Pain Prevention ... Head to Toe

Here are some acu-point tips to keep pain away throughout your day.

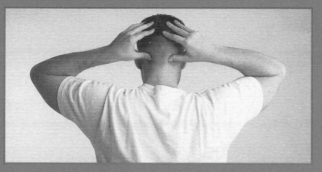

◄ For headaches in the back of the head or neck, use your thumbs to press firmly into GB-20 (Pool of Wind). Tilt your head up as you feel for the hollow spots on the back of your skull, located on either side of the spine. Use your fingers for support and stability while you gently press for two minutes. Breathe deeply.

➤ To ease bursitis of the shoulder, with thumb or reinforced index finger, press deeply into the joint with as much pressure as you can manage. Breathe deeply for 10 to 15 breaths as you slowly move the shoulder.

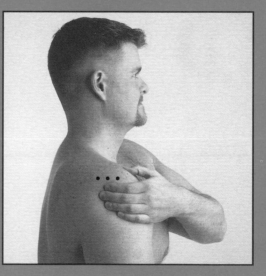

◄ Carpal tunnel syndrome need not cripple you with pain. While keeping your arm out straight and your hand in good alignment with your arm, pull straight back for 3 seconds, repeating 6–10 times while breathing deeply. A steady, gentle, even stretch of the carpal tunnel region will help relieve pain and tension. Repeat one or two times daily.

ALPHA

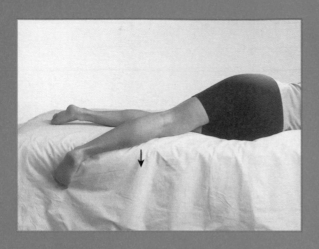

◁ To help relieve back pain, lie on an elevated table or bed. Let the top leg hang behind the lower leg. Breathe deeply and relax, allowing the weight of the leg to passively stretch the leg, hip, and low back.

▷Place a pillow under your knees and support your back by leaning against a wall. Find the tender spots on the outside crease of your knee (lateral meniscus) and inside (medial meniscus). Use your index and middle finger to press firmly for approximately one to two minutes per spot. Breathe deeply while rubbing vigorously with your palm afterwards.

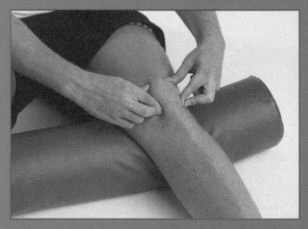

◁ For foot pain, while your leg is outstretched, wrap a towel around the top part of the foot. Breathe deeply as you pull straight back with even tension. Stretch for approximately 3 seconds at a time, pointing your foot for 6 or 10 repetitions. Repeat one or two times per day to relax tight tendons and get off on the right foot.

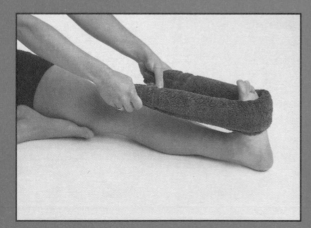

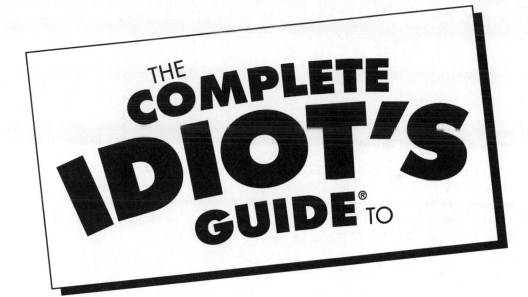

THE COMPLETE IDIOT'S GUIDE® TO

Acupuncture and Acupressure

by David Sollars

ALPHA

A member of Penguin Group (USA) Inc.

ALPHA BOOKS

Published by the Penguin Group

Penguin Group (USA) Inc., 375 Hudson Street, New York, New York 10014, U.S.A.

Penguin Group (Canada), 10 Alcorn Avenue, Toronto, Ontario, Canada M4V 3B2 (a division of Pearson Penguin Canada Inc.)

Penguin Books Ltd, 80 Strand, London WC2R 0RL, England

Penguin Ireland, 25 St Stephen's Green, Dublin 2, Ireland (a division of Penguin Books Ltd)

Penguin Group (Australia), 250 Camberwell Road, Camberwell, Victoria 3124, Australia (a division of Pearson Australia Group Pty Ltd)

Penguin Books India Pvt Ltd, 11 Community Centre, Panchsheel Park, New Delhi—110 017, India

Penguin Group (NZ), cnr Airborne and Rosedale Roads, Albany, Auckland 1310, New Zealand (a division of Pearson New Zealand Ltd)

Penguin Books (South Africa) (Pty) Ltd, 24 Sturdee Avenue, Rosebank, Johannesburg 2196, South Africa

Penguin Books Ltd, Registered Offices: 80 Strand, London WC2R 0RL, England

Copyright © 2000 by David Sollars

International Standard Book Number: 0-02-863942-1
Library of Congress Catalog Card Number: Available upon request.

07   06   05   8   7

Interpretation of the printing code: The rightmost number of the first series of numbers is the year of the book's printing; the rightmost number of the second series of numbers is the number of the book's printing. For example, a printing code of 00-1 shows that the first printing occurred in 2000.

Printed in the United States of America

Most Alpha books are available at special quantity discounts for bulk purchases for sales promotions, premiums, fund-raising, or educational use. Special books, or book excerpts, can also be created to fit specific needs.

For details, write: Special Markets, Alpha Books, 375 Hudson Street, New York, NY 10014.

Publisher
Marie Butler-Knight

Product Manager
Phil Kitchel

Managing Editor
Cari Luna

Senior Acquisitions Editor
Renee Wilmeth

Development Editor
Suzanne LeVert

Production Editor
JoAnna Kremer

Copy Editor
Amy Borrelli

Technical Editor
Amy Hull

Cover Designers
Mike Freeland
Kevin Spear

Book Designers
Scott Cook and Amy Adams of DesignLab

Indexer
Lisa Wilson

Layout/Proofreading
Darin Crone
Svetlana Dominguez
John Etchison
Mary Hunt
Bob LaRoche

Contents at a Glance

Table of Contents

Part 5: The Home Stretch 235

24 Expectations—Am I Better Yet? 237

25 Building a Winning Team 243

26 And Then There Was You—Taking Charge 249

Appendixes

Foreword

Just a generation ago, a Westerner suffering from a medical problem would consult the family doctor and, perhaps, an allopathic specialist. Today people can choose from among an explosion of treatments that extend beyond the bounds of conventional medicine. The consumer's challenge is to make sense of the interventions available and figure out which treatments—conventional, complementary, alternative or a combination of these—are likely to best heal their aches and pains and help them maintain good health.

"Oriental Medicine," which originated in China more than 2,000 years ago, is one "new" choice that is increasingly available in the West. At first glance, the treatments that belong under the heading of oriental medicine—acupuncture, acupressure, Chinese herbal medicine, qi gong—may seem exotic and mind boggling. Most of us need some guidance in navigating this complex medical system based on theories and terminology that can sound as foreign as the Chinese language itself.

That's where *The Complete Idiot's Guide to Acupuncture and Acupressure* comes in. In a single volume, David Sollars has succeeded in pulling together an accessible presentation of Oriental Medicine for the layperson. He clearly presents the medical theories on which acupuncture, acupressure, and its cousins are based, decodes key terminology, and straight-forwardly describes a variety of related treatments. Most important, he sheds light on the many medical conditions treatable by Oriental Medicine—from asthma to chronic pain to infertility and more.

At a time when Western civilization was still in its infancy, China had already developed this highly complex and effective medical system. Though known through the centuries to a small number of scholars, missionaries, and visitors to China, traditional Chinese medicine and its offshoots were, until recently, virtually unknown and unavailable in the West. Then with President Richard Nixon's widely publicized visit to China in 1973, ordinary Americans were introduced to acupuncture and oriental medicine. Within a few decades, this profound healing art has entered the mainstream.

Today the National Institutes of Health fund research in Oriental Medicine, more than 40 states license acupuncturists, and some insurance companies cover acupuncture services. Oriental Medical treatments, now available in conventional medical settings such as hospitals and community health centers, are used to treat an extensive range of conditions, some of which have been unresponsive to standard approaches. Accredited colleges of acupuncture and Oriental Medicine continue to spring up around the U.S. and abroad. And today we're even likely to hear a television character remark off-handedly about seeing an acupuncturist.

Despite the growing availability and acceptance of oriental medicine, too many people continue to suffer from illnesses and conditions, or undergo needless surgery, when acupuncture, acupressure, and related treatments could effectively and gently return them to health. This situation points to a need for more knowledge about Oriental Medicine on the part of patients and their Western-trained physicians. This simple yet comprehensive layman's guide will, I hope, encourage many more people to seek out Oriental Medicine to effectively heal illness and enhance well-being.

—Daniel D. Seitz, J.D.

President, New England School of Acupuncture; Chair, Accreditation Commission for Acupuncture and Oriental Medicine

Introduction

Those of us who practice oriental medicine have inherited a great legacy of healing arts that hold solutions for many of today's most stubborn and difficult health challenges. I have witnessed the rise in popularity of acupuncture, Chinese herbs, acupressure, and Qi Gong over my career, but this has not always meant that the general public truly understands this type of healing. I believe the potential contribution of oriental medicine lies in the ability of the modern-day practitioner to clearly and effectively educate our fellow healthcare providers, patients, and the general public about the unique and complementary therapies offered by an age-old system.

In striving to fully understand the foreign concepts and ideas behind oriental medicine, today's practitioners can help these therapies evolve by integrating them into our modern healthcare system. I envision a time when patients receive the best care possible, drawn from the various arenas of medicine. I am writing this book so that you get a glimpse of the system that I have been honored to study and share with my patients. Together we can help it evolve to better serve the needs of a world that strives for health and well-being.

How to Use This Book

For your convenience, this book is divided into five parts. You can move immediately to the conditions that affect you now, or browse the book to gain general insight into the practices featured. Since the best oriental medicine is based on individual evaluation and diagnosis, the explanations and advice given in this book are meant to be instructive, but cannot replace the proper care given by a qualified practitioner.

Statistically, most patients do not communicate with their conventional physicians about using traditional medicine. I encourage you to read these chapters, which include information in both therapies, so that you can be better informed about your condition and choices. Talk with your doctor and the people who are your health providers. This book is meant to be a bridge—be the first to step across!

Part 1 describes the basics of acupuncture and acupressure. Look here for theories about how energy moves through our bodies, and discover whether or not acupuncture hurts. By reading this section, you'll know what to expect on your first visit to the acu-pro, and you'll become familiar with the tools and techniques that are used to help you get well.

Parts 2 through **4** cover conditions for which acupuncture and acupressure appear to be most helpful. By using oriental medicine, you'll greatly alleviate those conditions as well as improve your overall health. **Part 5** will help you put your knowledge into practice by showing you how to pick a qualified acu-pro and build your healthcare team. We'll discuss what to expect from your treatment and how your own contributions will lead you toward health and peace of mind.

At the end of the book, I include a glossary of terms concerning acupuncture, as well as a host of resources that will allow you to expand your knowledge of oriental medicine and help you find the most qualified oriental health professionals in your area. I hope you will enjoy reading this book, and that it will be the beginning of a new approach to health and freedom.

Acu-Boxes for Accurate Understanding

Throughout the book, you'll find boxes that contain valuable tips for treatment and for better understanding of oriental medicine.

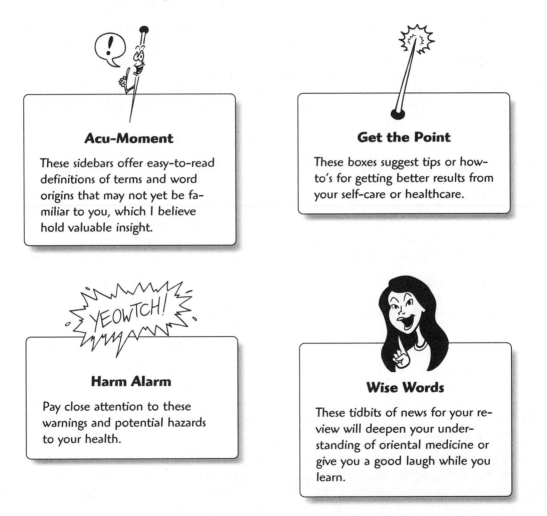

Acu-Moment

These sidebars offer easy-to-read definitions of terms and word origins that may not yet be familiar to you, which I believe hold valuable insight.

Get the Point

These boxes suggest tips or how-to's for getting better results from your self-care or healthcare.

Harm Alarm

Pay close attention to these warnings and potential hazards to your health.

Wise Words

These tidbits of news for your review will deepen your understanding of oriental medicine or give you a good laugh while you learn.

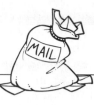

Mailbag

These sidebars contain real-life anecdotes from my patients about their experiences with acupuncture and acupressure. You will get a glimpse of the conditions they came in with, the techniques we used, the frequency of office visits, and the final outcome.

Acknowledgments

This book—or any book on oriental medicine—would not be possible to produce in English without the talented and dedicated work of Oriental Medical translators. Their pursuit of knowledge and desire to share the wealth of accumulated medical expertise, which has been evolving in Oriental Medicine over the past three centuries, benefits the many educators and practitioners around the world. I was fortunate in being able to study with some of the best practitioners. Their high standards and caring have inspired me to strive for that mix of art form and medical skills.

I am grateful to have studied with Andy Gamble, Kiku Miyazaki, Lea and Tom Tam, Ping Chuan, and Dr. Yang Jwing Ming. Our profession is constantly recreating itself to fulfill the challenges of a new century of healthcare. Acupuncture and acupressure schools and organizations continue to foster excitement and expertise in new practitioners. They are the guardians of our standards.

I want to thank the New England School of Acupuncture for giving me a solid foundation in Oriental Medicine. I have also gained a lot of knowledge from working with my fellow practitioners; I am in awe of the talented health providers in this field and am grateful to continue learning from my peers. I also want to acknowledge the knowledge I gain from my patients. I am grateful to be a part of so many families' lives This profession allows me to know and appreciate the people who come to see me and entrust me with the care of their families and friends.

Thanks to Laura Lavensaller: I am grateful for her initial groundwork, which helped shape the possibility of this book.

I certainly want to thank Alpha Books and the team of editors who believed in this book and helped me make it possible. Your patience and expertise have allowed me to write from my head and my heart. Thank you Renee, Suzanne, JoAnna, and Amy.

Special thanks to the models of this book: Diane, Heather, and Kern. And thanks to Stuart and Jane for allowing Lauren's talented participation.

Finally, my family has put up with my rigorous schedules and has supported and encouraged me to reach for the stars. My parents always let me know they believed in me, even if they didn't quite understand what I was doing. Laura, my sister-in-law and fellow acupuncturist, provided the initial inspiration for this book. My stepchildren, Heather and Shawn, have given me acceptance and love, and taught me more about life than any university I have attended! My wife, Diane, has been the best life partner I could have hoped for. She welcomed me into her family with sparkling magic and dove-cooing love. She has worked side-by-side with me as I wrote this book, acting as an editor, adviser, and round-the-clock coach.

Special Thanks to the Technical Reviewer

The Complete Idiot's Guide to Acupuncture and Acupressure was reviewed by an expert who double-checked the accuracy of what you'll learn here, to help us ensure that this book gives you everything you need to know about this aspect of oriental medicine. Special thanks are extended to Amy Hull. She was not only my classmate through acupuncture school, but has inspired me by her dedication to sharing her knowledge with others as a professor and as Assistant Dean of Education at The New England School of Acupuncture. Thank you for being the technical editor for this book. You contributed valuable suggestions and insights.

Trademarks

All terms mentioned in this book that are known to be or are suspected of being trademarks or service marks have been appropriately capitalized. Alpha Books and Penguin Group (USA) Inc. cannot attest to the accuracy of this information. Use of a term in this book should not be regarded as affecting the validity of any trademark or service mark.

Part 1

From Mystery to Miracles

What are acupuncture and acupressure, and how do they work? We'll look at the distant roots of these popular point therapies to see what makes them tick.

This section also takes the mystery out of your first visit to an acupuncture professional by letting you know what to expect. You'll discover the information your acu-pro needs in order to assist you in putting together an effective treatment plan. From looking and listening to pressing and poking, it's all here to help you open your mind. You'll begin your journey through some of the most fascinating and empowering healing techniques of all time … well, maybe just the last four or five thousand years!

Chapter 1

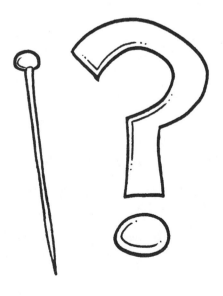

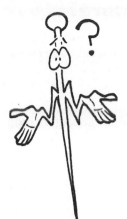

What Are Acupuncture and Acupressure, and How Do They Work?

In This Chapter

➤ What are acupuncture and acupressure?

➤ What are acu-points and how can you find them?

➤ How it all works

➤ Puncture or pressure: similarities and differences

When my patients respond favorably from undergoing acupuncture and acupressure therapies, they almost always look surprised and ask two questions: "Why didn't I do this sooner?" and "How on earth does this stuff work?" This chapter begins to answer that second question by giving you an overview of these ancient healing arts that have become so popular in today's growing field of alternative/complementary medicine. You'll learn the ancient principles of oriental *Qi* (*chee*) flow and the current explanations of how it works in your body. You'll discover that you, too, have energy channels and acu-points, and I'll show you how to find them like the pros do. By the end of the chapter, you'll know when to use acupuncture or acupressure and when not to.

There's no need to answer the first question ("Why didn't I do this sooner?"), because it's never too late. Keep turning these pages and learn for yourself the benefits of these dynamic healing arts.

What Are Acupuncture and Acupressure?

You've probably already seen acupuncture featured on a television show or in a newspaper or magazine article. I'm encouraged to see it's even made it into the comic strips! It tells me that acupuncture has become part of our culture, which means that whether you've used it or not, you most likely have images in your mind about what it is. You may even know someone who has tried it.

The National Institutes of Health's consensus statement from its November 1997 conference states: "Acupuncture describes a family of procedures involving stimulation of anatomical locations on the skin by a variety of techniques. There are a variety of approaches that incorporate medical traditions from China, Japan, Korea, and other countries."

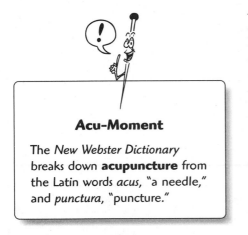

Acu-Moment

The *New Webster Dictionary* breaks down **acupuncture** from the Latin words *acus*, "a needle," and *punctura*, "puncture."

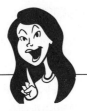

Wise Words

The word **meridian** is often used in place of channels in many oriental medical books. Its French origin refers to pathways that encircle our earth, which compare to the channels that encircle our bodies.

Acupuncture is part of a complete system of diagnosis and treatments in oriental medicine. In acupuncture, health is maintained by the smooth flow of life energy—or Qi— through pathways in our bodies called channels or meridians. Channels act as conduits or pipes that maintain balance and health throughout our body's skin, muscles, and organs. They're like the pipes in your home supplying heat and water so that your home can function smoothly. If a pipe becomes clogged, you've got problems. When injuries, emotions, disease, stress, or poor lifestyle choices disrupt the circulation of qi, blood, lymph, and other fluids in your body, you begin to feel worse and medical symptoms appear.

Acupressure is the gentle but firm stimulation of acupoints by fingers, thumbs, elbows, and even feet. The same points are used along the energy channels as in acupuncture, but acupressure is carried out without the use of needles. Acupressure is part of Oriental Medicine and has developed several unique styles of diagnosis and treatment throughout the world (see Chapter 3, "The Origins of Oriental Medicine").

Energy Channels: Go with the Flow

Imagine a series of invisible pipes, canals, or even hallways that begin within your skin and connect to every tissue and organ inside your body. According to traditional oriental medicine, these channels—or *meridians*—transport your life's energy, or Qi, along with blood and bodily fluids that nourish and moisten your entire system. It's a two-way street from the outside to the inside, transporting diseases or the healing stimulation of acu-points. With so much traffic along these pathways, you can see why it's vital to your health to keep them running smoothly and efficiently. In fact, illness results from the traffic jams in your channels. This disruption in flow may occur just where you feel it, or may be the result of a problem "upstream" in another part of your body. Your acu-pro, a term I use throughout this text to identify a practitioner who uses either acupressure or acupuncture, will help you determine the origin of the blockage and assist you in unblocking it.

Acu-Points: Mini but Mighty

The Chinese meaning of "acupuncture point" is the combination of the words "hole" and "position." These points serve as external doors or openings to the channels that access the internal muscles and organs of your body. No one knows exactly how these points' healing properties were discovered, but the earliest written document dates back to *The Yellow Emperor's Inner Classic* (second century B.C.E.). By then, points had been assigned to a channel according to similar curative benefits and given names describing what they were used for. Also, a numbering system was developed to match their order of placement on the channel. For instance, ST-36 (the Three Mile Point) is on the stomach channel and is the 36th point of the channel. This point is used for a wide variety of stomach complaints as well as general energy, hence the traditional name indicating this point will give your legs three more miles worth of energy.

You can locate acu-points on main channels that traverse your body up, down, and sideways. Most of the 361 main channel points had been identified by the third century C.E.

But the Chinese didn't stop there. Other points were discovered in the ear that could affect corresponding muscles or organs. In fact, new points are continually being discovered in China, and in many countries where acupuncture is widely practiced. New uses for existing points are being developed as the integration of conventional western medicine and traditional oriental medicine progresses. These points may be found by electro-conductivity testing of skin or measuring the microcurrents that exist where channels and nerve trunks intersect. (You'll know more about what I'm talking about here when you read the section later in this chapter, "How Does It Work— The Key to the Qi.") Keep pressing your points and perhaps you'll discover a new one yourself!

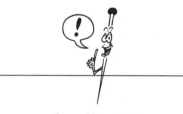

Acu-Moment

An **Ah Shi** point, developed by Sun Si Mao (581–682 C.E.), is any point that is sore when pressed. On or off the channels, it may be used as a special point or indicator to diagnose or treat a condition.

Finding Your Points—Come Out, Come Out, Wherever You Are!

Acu-points are typically, but not always found in the valleys of muscles and joints. They are often sensitive to finger pressure, especially when a point reflects an illness or condition that is present in your body. Your acu-pro has spent many hours memorizing the locations of these points, but how does he or she find them on you?

Anatomy: The Thigh Bone's Connected to the ...

You can find acu-points anywhere on your body by using proportional measurements of anatomy. Equal measurements of each part of the body by a system of unit measurements help to locate acu-points relative to the physical proportions of the individual. No matter how big or small your arm is, it's divided into 12 units from shoulder to elbow and 9 units from elbow to wrist (see the following figure).

Unit measurements simplify your search.

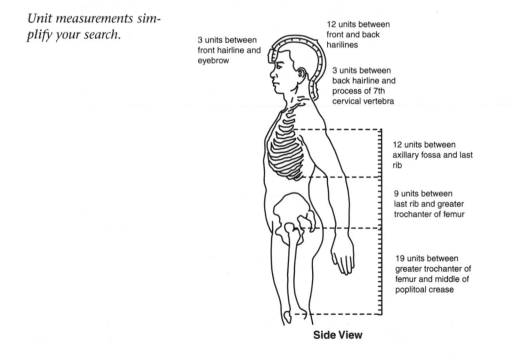

3 units between front hairline and eyebrow

12 units between front and back harilines

3 units between back hairline and process of 7th cervical vertebra

12 units between axillary fossa and last rib

9 units between last rib and greater trochanter of femur

19 units between greater trochanter of femur and middle of poplitoal crease

Side View

Finger Measurements: Let Your Fingers Do the Walking

The physical landmarks and units get you in the right neighborhood; using more precise finger units will put you on the spot.

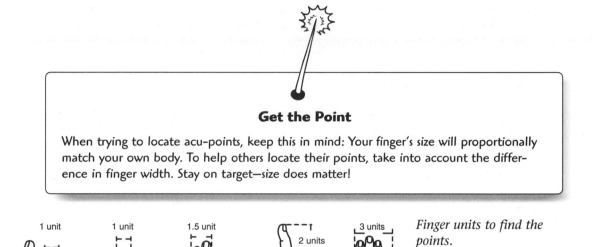

Get the Point

When trying to locate acu-points, keep this in mind: Your finger's size will proportionally match your own body. To help others locate their points, take into account the difference in finger width. Stay on target—size does matter!

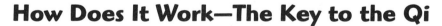

Finger units to find the points.

How Does It Work—The Key to the Qi

Take a minute and rub your hands vigorously together. Now pull them apart slightly and feel the warmth and tingling between your hands. Pull them apart even farther and notice that you still feel sensations. Theories of Qi in our body have been used to explain experiences like what you've just felt. Ancient oriental philosophers and physicians sought to understand why people got sick and what kept them well. They noticed a myriad of environmental and bodily sensations that seemed to reoccur in distinctive patterns over and over again. Such sensations as warmth, relaxation, and tingling have all been attributed to healthy Qi flow and are the same sensations you'll experience when stimulating your acu-points.

Bioelectric Flow: What's the Buzz All About?

Since the early 1950s, scientists have noticed a peculiar phenomenon with acu-points. Electrical properties of the skin along channels and points are different than nonchannel or point locations. If an organ is removed or the tissue crossed by the channel is destroyed, the electrical potential decreases, even disappears. Scientists have observed consistent characteristics of an independent electrical conduit in the body. This conduit works with the nervous system but does not follow all of its rules. This suggests a separate system of circulating energy that is different yet interactive with the nervous and cardiovascular systems that have been well observed and studied in conventional medicine.

This interaction or communication between the acupoints, channels, and corresponding muscles and organs of our body is at the heart of understanding how Qi flows and heals. While no perfect study or explanation exists, the majority of practitioners agree that the electrical conductivity model explains what makes the system measurable to scientists.

Electrical phenomena are usually measured in two ways. The first method applies electrical current to the skin and then scientists measure electro conductivity and resistance to gauge the difference between an acu-point or channel and an area off the path. The second method applies no external source of electricity, but instead takes measurements on the surface of the skin to gauge its own electrical potential. Some changes in the skin's electrical currents have been shown to correspond to the internal organs that the channels are connected with. New developments in research will allow practitioners and scientists to create more meaningful study models for evaluating and understanding if electrical phenomena are the best way to identify the mechanism of acu-points and channels.

Biomagnetic Flow Pulls You to the Point

Our bodies are also made up of measurable magnetic fields. Practitioners demonstrate this by placing biomagnets on the acu-points and measuring the microcurrents in the nerves that increase blood flow. Researchers have been busy explaining why magnets, which are all the rage, seem to help so many people feel better.

There are a multitude of magnetic therapy products available, but the science behind their efficacy is still poorly understood. The Qi channels seem to respond to magnetic stimulation. Because there is a growing amount of clinical anecdotal case studies that reflect benefits—and I have seen this in my own patients—it is my guess that that reliable research will be coming to our industry. Japan has been a main contributor of research so far, but other countries and industry are following.

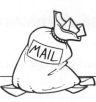

Mailbag

Ellen was 39 years of age and had been working as an artist for 15 years. At the time, she was designing and making her own line of earrings and pins. She came in to see me complaining of low back pain from a recent overnight work session to get ready for a trade show. She could barely walk, was stooped over with acute pain, and had to twist her body to the side and lift her head in order to say hello for our first meeting. Her friends had seen me before for similar complaints and had suggested she come for treatment. She explained that this would probably not work because she was a "doctor's daughter" and didn't really "believe in this stuff," but was so desperate she'd try anything. I proceeded to give her a treatment of needle acupuncture followed by acupressure and stretching. At each step her pain diminished and her mood became friendlier and less combative. By the end of the session she was walking upright, and had several exercises to continue at home. I explained she didn't need to "believe," just be open for change.

Different Yet the Same

We've seen how acupuncture and acupressure use the same channels and points. In addition, they use many of the same diagnostic principles in oriental medicine and hope to aid you in achieving the same quality of health by balancing the qi in your body. Acupuncturists may use needles, which they are more famous for, but they also have a variety of instruments that we'll explore further in Chapter 5, "Acupuncture—Tools of the Trade." Acupressure therapists use everything from their fingers to their feet. Which will be best for you? The enjoyment of finding the answer to these questions will lead you to the talented acu-pros in your area. Soon you'll discover what combination works best for you.

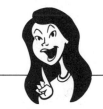

Wise Words

Watch where you apply pressure. Staying on the point makes all the difference. Research demonstrates that the effects of stimulating acu-points are pronounced, while non-acu sites are either weak or nonexistent.

Healthcare Versus Self-Care

Whether you see an acupuncturist, an acupressurist, or your family physician, you're asking someone to assist you with your healthcare, which means you want to find a qualified, caring health professional. His or her training and experience will aid you and your family by the use of many tools and techniques. In self-care, your acu-pro educates and instructs you in the acupressure, exercise, or lifestyle changes that will either speed up your healing or keep you on track to continue feeling good. Both parts are essential in maintaining your optimal health.

Congratulations! You've learned that you too, have Qi running through you body and can hopefully begin to visualize how it's distributed through channels that interconnect your skin with your muscles, nerves, and organs. You can also start using the oriental finger measurements called "cun" to locate the points you'll be learning to use in the rest of the book. I've also introduced the important concept of healthcare and self-care that we'll discuss throughout this text so that you'll not only learn how an acu-pro can help, but also what you can do yourself to be active in the healing process. In the next chapter, you'll learn what it's like to visit an acu-pro and separate fact from fiction.

The Least You Need to Know

➤ Qi is often experienced as a warm, tingling, heavy sensation followed by relaxation.

➤ Acu-points are the doorways that lead in and out of your body.

➤ Finding acu-points is easy with unit measurements and finger widths.

➤ Bioelectric and biomagnetic theories do not fully explain how acu-points work to heal, but are a good start.

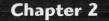

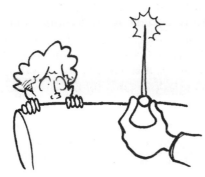

Chapter 2

What to Expect on Your First Visit— Does It Hurt?

In This Chapter

➤ See your tongue in a whole new light

➤ Your pulse will tell you more than your just heartbeat

➤ Discover why acupuncture doesn't hurt

➤ Learn when *not* to go for treatment

➤ Relax and enjoy the ride

You're thinking of going for an acupuncture or acupressure treatment, but are hesitant or even skeptical. You don't know what's going to happen, so you keep putting it off: *"Maybe tomorrow I'll call for an appointment."* You're not alone. While the popularity of these therapies is growing, most of your friends and family have not gone for treatment … yet.

In this chapter, you'll learn what kind of information about you and your health that your acu-pro needs in order to figure out how to help you. Knowing what to expect takes most of the mystery and anxiety out of your first visit, so that you can concentrate on your health. Afterwards, you'll feel great and wonder what all the fuss was about.

Looking: Mirror, Mirror on the Wall

The first thing your acu-pro will do is look at your general appearance and vitality. Are you a vibrant, assertive person with plenty of outward energy, or do you come across as weak and frail? These are the first general observations that he or she will make. Your body type may also be noted. If you are overweight, you're more likely to be affected by illnesses stemming from disorders of dampness, while being too thin means you might be prone to imbalances of yin energies (see Chapter 6, "How You Get Sick—The Good, the Bad, and the Ugly").

Your acu-pro will also observe your posture, skin tone, and texture of your face. If you have a chalky, bloated face, it can often mean that your Qi (life energy) is low, most likely stemming from poor digestion. A black or dark color under the eyes points to a deficiency in kidney energy, either in the organ itself or somewhere along the pathways of its related energy channels. It's worth mentioning that channels and their organs often share the same name, which reflects their interconnectedness. In Oriental Medical terminology, for instance, kidney energy may refer to the channel of Qi that runs along the kidney channel as well as the energy in the kidney organ itself. Your acu-pro will most likely be discussing the channel he or she is working on and not the organ. If there's any confusion, just ask.

Tongue Diagnosis: Open Wide and Say "Aaah!"

The tongue is an important part of oriental medical diagnosis. The tongue is connected to many of the Qi channels and reflects the organs that the channels pass through. Take a minute and go to your bathroom mirror and stick out your tongue. Notice the size, shape, and color of your tongue, and remember to look at the fuzzy layer on top. Also look for any cracks or bumps along the sides, tip, or surface of the tongue. A normal tongue should be pinkish, with a slight, thin, white coating that has no bumps or teeth marks along the sides. It may make us sound like we're fortune-tellers, but this is a sophisticated medical system that acupuncturists have been using clinically for thousands of years.

A tongue with a thin, red tip usually indicates two things. One, it could be a pizza burn. The second—and more likely—possibility is that you're experiencing a great deal of anxiety or some emotional burden. A red tip suggests that the emotions have gotten stuck and could be affecting your body and mind with repetitive thoughts, insomnia, or dream-disturbed sleep. It's a good idea to take a look at your tongue periodically. Your tongue reflects the state of health in general and specific ways. It will begin to change even with the onset of a cold. Your acu-pro will share his or her observation with you so you can keep an eye on things yourself.

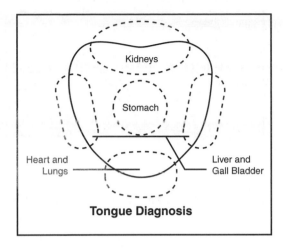

Tongue diagnosis.

Tongue Diagnosis

- Kidneys
- Stomach
- Heart and Lungs
- Liver and Gall Bladder

Your Pulse: Feel the Beat

Your conventional physician checks your heart rate by taking your pulse. By pressing on the radial artery located where the wrist meets your hand, he or she can determine the number of times per minute your heart beats. In Oriental Medicine, your pulse gives clues to the condition of the channels that run over your body and your corresponding organs. Although each channel has its own pulse points located on the body, the three pulse positions located on each wrist are traditionally the principle sites for pulse diagnosis. Your acu-pro must feel and distinguish between three pulse positions with three depths to each position. Right now, as you are reading, place one of your wrists in the palm of the other hand (see the following figure). Let's begin your first pulse-reading exercise.

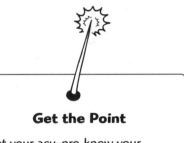

Get the Point

Let your acu-pro know your habits. Brushing your tongue with your toothbrush; drinking tea, coffee, or grape juice; or sucking on cinnamon candy may change the coating and color of your tongue. To avoid confusion, let your acu–pro know what you last ate or drank.

Wrap your fingers around your wrist so that the tips of your index, middle, and ring fingers lightly touch the outside edge of the underside of the wrist. Do you feel the beat? What else do you feel? Does it feel strong or weak? Does it remind you of a tight guitar string or a limp noodle? These subtle characteristics are what your acu-pro is trained to detect when taking your pulses. While pulse diagnosis is used in conjunction with the other diagnostic procedures in this chapter, a skilled practitioner can often tell a great deal about your condition from your pulse readings alone.

Checking your pulse the oriental way.

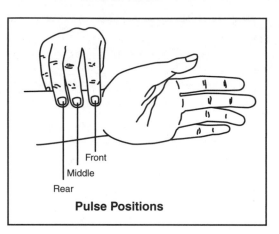

Front
Middle
Rear

Pulse Positions

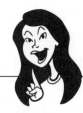

Wise Words

My, your lungs are busy. One inhalation and one exhalation are called one **respiration.** Your pulse beats four times in one respiration. The average person has between 24,000– 26,000 respirations per day. Athletes are typically slower, while children are faster.

A slow, short, weak, slippery middle pulse (on the right hand) often indicates trapped cold in your body with insufficient Qi in the digestive system. A slippery quality, which feels like a thick liquid squishing under your fingertips, indicates that dampness has interrupted the smooth flow of Qi in your stomach (see Chapter 6), and you may have a sluggish digestion, excess mucus, and/or heaviness of limbs. All this from your pulse? See your acu-pro and find out even more that lies behind the beating of your pulse.

Listening and Asking: The Hidden Arts

An old adage states that you were given two ears and one mouth so you could listen twice as much. The truth of that statement is even more ringing in Oriental Medicine. Your practitioner will certainly take a thorough medical history from you, cover your symptoms, and want to know your preferences for hot or cold drinks and food desires. Sounds like he or she is preparing the perfect meal for you! In reality, however, your acu-pro wants to understand how you experience health and illness. Everything from how you digest food to your sleeping patterns gives more information and proper perspective to your condition.

Your practitioner must also listen. He or she will focus on your speech and breathing patterns and listen to your cough or wheeze. A cough that gurgles is due to phlegm or dampness, while a dry hacking cough relates to dry heat trapped in the lungs (see Chapter 6). These sounds are helpful information your practitioner uses to compile an oriental medical diagnosis and create a successful treatment plan, which is very important because the practitioner will treat these conditions very differently.

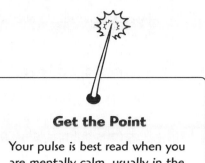

Get the Point

Your pulse is best read when you are mentally calm, usually in the early morning or a few minutes after arriving at work. Traditionally, you should read your pulse on both wrists while keeping your hands below the level of your heart.

Smelling: Pass the Perfume

The nose may know a thing or two. Excessive heat conditions in the lungs, stomach, or bowels produce very foul breath or body odors. Excessive cold illnesses have a distinctive rotten fish smell. Hmmm, just what I like to experience right after lunch! I have often heard patients say they can smell when they are getting sick. Different odors are associated with specific organ systems, and often patients' individual odors vanish as their health improves.

Today, perfumes and deodorant soaps cover up many of these significant odors that a few centuries ago would be obvious to anyone within whiffing distance! So a strong smell that reaches out to you is usually significant to the condition. Your practitioner will keep up his or her snoopy sniffing; after all, the nose knows!

Physical Exam: Follow the Yellow Brick Road

Another part of your initial visit will be for your acu-pro to closely examine the condition of your channels, points, muscles, and joints. Soreness of acu-points and channels can generate helpful information about the corresponding muscles or organ systems that the channel crosses. Take a moment to check for yourself.

Check Your Channels

Here's a way to check one part of your body to see how well (or poorly) the Qi is flowing. If you are pregnant, however, don't use this test because it influences the lower abdomen. (However, locating this acu-point may prove helpful later in your pregnancy because it can be stimulated to induce labor for an easy delivery. See Chapter 16, "Birthing Baby.")

➤ Place the four fingers of your hand on the inside of your ankle.

➤ Lay the little finger at the tip of the inside of the anklebone.

➤ Press the point in the middle of the soft part of the leg next to your index finger (this point is SP-6, Three Yin Crossing).

➤ Press gently but firmly around this point and feel if there's an achy or soft spot.

➤ Follow this channel by gently pressing the inside of your leg to the knee.

Check the channels of your leg with firm, gentle, pressure.

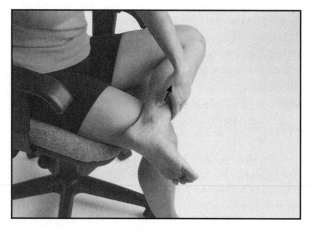

Soreness of this point and channel represent the muscles and tendons on the inside of the leg, but can also detect imbalances in the lower abdomen. This might be particularly sore if you were experiencing difficulties with constipation, PMS, chronic bladder infections, or bloating.

If your main complaints include a muscular-skeletal problem, such as bursitis in your shoulder or back pain, expect to have pressure sensitivity on those muscles and joints evaluated and written down. Other physical examinations, such as range of motion, may be performed to see if your natural movement is restricted in any way.

Your acu-pro is trained to understand the relationship between the nerves, muscles, tendons, and ligaments in your body. A thorough exam will help both of you judge the progress of future treatments.

Abdomen: The Bounty of the Belly

You may have had your abdomen, the area below your ribs and above the pubic bone, checked by your physician when you were pregnant or if you complained of stomach or bowel problems. To your acu-pro, however, the abdomen holds a bounty of information about your current state of health. Many of your Qi channels cross over your belly, and gentle pressure applied to specific areas will help confirm your practitioner's thoughts about your condition.

Is This Safe?

Acupuncture and acupressure are both almost risk free as therapies. There are no side effects such as we find with drug therapy, and the safety records in this country and internationally help to explain why these methods have become so popular. Let's take a look.

Acupressure: Press Safely!

Acupressure uses your body as its only tool. As long as the pressure is applied in a gentle manner, there are few safety considerations. Acupressure is safe to receive, use as a self-care treatment, or share with your family and friends. Some cautions to remember include the following:

➤ Apply firm, gentle pressure; avoid pressing in a quick, jarring, or forceful manner.

➤ Do not apply pressure to a burn, ulcer, or infection.

➤ Avoid abdominal pressure if you are pregnant or have medical illnesses such as colon cancer, leukemia, or a serious cardiac condition.

➤ Avoid applying pressure to recently formed scar tissue around an operation or injury for the first month of healing. Points that are several inches away, however, can be used to help speed up your recovery.

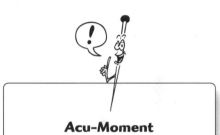

Acu-Moment

The National Certification for the Commission of Acupuncture and Oriental Medicine (NC-CAOM) was established in 1984 to set national standards in the United States. It has certified over 9,000 acupuncturists and has never had reason to take action due to negligent or harmful treatment of a patient.

Acupuncture: The Safer the Better

Evidence clearly shows that acupuncture is very safe when performed by a well-trained practitioner. In China and Japan, where millions of treatments take place every year, only 10 injuries have been reported since 1972. In the United States, 10 injuries have been reported since 1965. This compares with nearly one million injuries in this country caused by conventional medical procedures and drug side effects in just one single year.

There are specific cautions and contraindications listed in Chapter 5, "Acupuncture—Tools of the Trade," for each acupuncture technique. In general, here are a few points to remember:

➤ Your pregnancy can be greatly improved with acupuncture, but not all points are used, such as abdominal and low back.

➤ Avoid acupuncture in open wounds, ulcers, or undiagnosed swellings.

➤ Avoid electricity attached to the needles if you have a pacemaker or serious heart condition.

➤ Let your acupuncturist know if you are weak or woozy from fatigue or hunger.

➤ You should not have acupuncture if you are intoxicated or taking recreational drugs.

The profession also developed *The Clean Needle Technique Manual* in conjunction with the Centers for Disease Control in Atlanta, Georgia. This manual serves as a basis for the courses, both written and practical, which are required to pass the NC-CAOM certification and for licensure in most states. All of these steps ensure that you see qualified practitioners when seeking help through Oriental Medicine.

Your Treatment: Relax and Enjoy

You're finished with all the talking. Now it's time to lay back and let the healing begin.

The Power of Pleasing Pressure

Acupressure is often performed while you are fully clothed, either on a massage table or a soft, comfortable floor mat. Treatments consist of a firm but gentle pressure applied to acu-points by the practitioner's fingers, thumbs, elbows, knees, or feet. You will always be asked if the pressure is comfortable. The treatment may last from one to two hours, depending on the style of the practitioner and the goals you have set. Gentle stretching of your muscles and channels may also be part of your experience.

There may also be soft music playing to help you relax and unwind. I have found that deep breathing is particularly effective in conjunction with acupressure to melt away sore muscles and go into a deep, relaxed state. I often suggest some deep-breathing exercises to my patients during the treatment sessions.

Acupuncture: The Painless Truth

If you've never experienced acupuncture, you probably have one overriding question: "Does it hurt?" It's estimated that 12 million Americans made visits to acupuncturists in 1993; this number has most likely tripled by now. How could that be if it hurts so much? The truth is, it doesn't hurt at all. When you go in for your first acupuncture treatment, you'll soon realize (as have all of my patients) that the insertion of the hairlike needle is either completely unnoticed by you, or you merely feel a slight pinch.

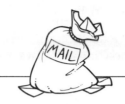

Mailbag

Helen worked as an executive secretary with much of her day spent doing keyboard and mouse work. She was in a high-pressure job where performance counts, and the growing discomfort in her wrists and arms worried her. She tried the usual route of anti-inflammatory medications and a course of physical therapy without the desired results. She continued to worry. I met her almost a year after her pain began. Although friends urged her to try acupuncture, she'd been afraid that the needles would hurt. Following her first treatment, however, she was pleasantly relieved to have a painless experience and was embarrassed at how long she waited to come for help. Acupuncture and acupressure techniques helped ease Helen's discomfort and, like many other patients, she found out any sensations she may experience during the course of treatment are well worth the results they bring.

Now that you know it doesn't hurt, let's see what really does happen at an acupuncture treatment session. Your acupuncturist will have you lie on a comfortable massage-like treatment table. Depending on the areas to be worked on, you may need to roll up your sleeves or pant legs, or use a gown or sheet as a partial cover-up, similar to what you are accustomed to at your conventional physician's office. The number of needles to be inserted depends on your condition and the style of practice your acupuncturist performs (see Chapter 3, "The Origins of Oriental Medicine").

Typical sensations during acupuncture range from no feeling at all, to soothing warmth, to tingling, to electrical "buzzing," to a dull ache. These are all normal responses and will vary depending on each individual's condition and your practitioner's techniques. Your acupuncturist can stimulate each point in a way that is best suited to treat your condition.

Some needles are inserted very shallow under the skin, while others may need to be in the belly of the muscle or joint. Wherever the needles need to go, your practitioner is skilled in making your experience safe, effective, and comfortable. Your first visit may include the use of some other techniques, like heat or massage (see Chapter 5).

Treatment time averages from one-half hour to one hour. If the acupuncturist decides to leave the needles in place for a time, it's usually for about 20 minutes to half an hour. Often, you'll listen to soothing music to help you relax.

During acupuncture or acupressure, your body releases endorphins, which are natural painkillers, and serotonin, a feel-good brain chemical. Circulation increases and your body's systems are helped to let go of stress and function more normally. This chemical release helps explain the powerful effects of these therapies. Depending on your particular condition, you may be asked to avoid heavy meals of meats or starches, excessive exercise, alcohol, or sex for 12–24 hours after treatment. These may work counterproductive to your treatment. Allowing your body to continue balancing without strong stimulants may improve the success of your visits. Make sure you wrap up and stay warm. During treatment, you body temperature often lowers; pores and circulation are now open, temporarily making you more vulnerable to the elements.

Following your first visit, you now have bragging rights and can share with your family and friends what it's like to experience these dynamic healing arts.

Now that you have an idea what a visit to your acu-pro will be like, read on and find out how this all got started. You may be surprised how it all came together.

The Least You Need to Know

➤ Facial skin tone and texture reflect organ health.

➤ Teeth marks around your tongue suggest poor digestion.

➤ Pressing your pulse and abdomen unlocks clues to your condition.

➤ Excessive heat trapped in your lungs or stomach produces foul breath.

➤ Acupuncture and acupressure are safe and comfortable when performed by qualified practitioners.

Chapter 3

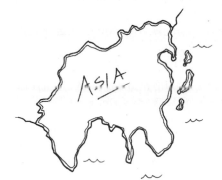

The Origins of Oriental Medicine

In This Chapter

➤ How medicine merged in China over 2,000 years ago

➤ Acupressure choices to pick from

➤ The many faces of acupuncture

➤ The acu-life goes global

The term "Oriental Medicine" is itself too simplistic when it comes to describing a vast body of medical knowledge that has endured over several thousand years. Many eastern countries, including India and Japan, added their own distinct advances in theory and techniques. Indeed, acupuncture and acupressure have their roots in the traditions of medicine that began in China over 3,000 years ago and have spread throughout the world ever since. We'll explore its fascinating history in this chapter.

Acupuncture: The Ancient Art

In the beginning, early practitioners turned to observing nature in an attempt to figure out why some people got sick on a cold rainy day and others didn't. They observed the changes of the seasons and the effects they had on men and women, physically and emotionally.

With nature playing such a large role, it isn't surprising that different regions of China played different roles in medical development. In the northern part of China (the Yellow River district), for instance, the soil is infertile. There are many rocks and boulders, and plants are limited to small grasses. When people were injured, they used wood and stone splinters to pick out infection. Another popular technique that developed in this cold region was warming specific points of the body by placing one of the small grass plants, dried mugwort (see Chapter 5, "Acupuncture—Tools of the Trade"), and lighting it on fire. (Kids, don't try this at home!) They found that the heat gave relief to many health problems caused by too much cold in the environment. Doesn't this help you appreciate your central heating system?

The tradition of acupressure grew out of the habit of pressing and rubbing chilled or numb areas of the body with fingers or palms of the hand. Through practice, the northern Chinese developed effective techniques, including stimulating points on the body with finger-pressure, pieces of stone, and burning herbs.

In southern China, the weather is warmer (Yangtze River district) and the land is rich with plants of all kinds. When these folks got sick, they also used what was available from their environment. Twigs, bark, and roots from this region became the foundation of Chinese herbal medicine.

Archeologists have found acupuncture needles and medical information written on bones from as far back as the Shang Dynasty (1000 B.C.E.). The northern and southern styles of medicine were finally combined through trade, travel, and war during the Han Dynasty (220 C.E.). By the fourth century C.E., a relatively sophisticated medicine existed in China that used acupuncture channel theory, herbs, and acupressure, and had complex theories to explain how you got sick and what to do to feel better.

As it is today, medical knowledge was always quite valuable. Chinese medicine continued to evolve as it spread through Korea, Japan, and other eastern countries. Due to the nature of the land and the medical problems they dealt with, each country added new thoughts and treatments to the collection of customs accumulated along the way.

In the United States, especially during the latter half of the twentieth century, we combined all traditions under the rubric of "Oriental Medicine."

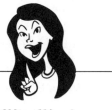

Wise Words

A Short History of Medicine

"Doctor, I have an earache."
2000 B.C.E.—"Here, eat this root."
1000 B.C.E.—"That root is heathen, say this prayer."
1850 C.E.—"That prayer is superstition, drink this potion."
1940 C.E.—"That potion is snake oil, swallow this pill."
1985 C.E.—"That pill is ineffective, take this antibiotic."
2000 C.E.—"That antibiotic is artificial. Here, eat this root!"

Types of Acupressure: Choices, Choices, and More Choices

Most countries have a tradition of some form of massage or acupressure. It's a natural instinct to rub an area that is sore or tired. Acupressure therapists may be called numerous names, depending on the country or medical theories that influenced their growth.

For starters, we'll discuss two of my favorites.

Shiatsu

Shiatsu (*she-aht-sue*) is a popular form of Japanese acupressure. *Shi* means "finger," and *atsu* means "pressure." Shiatsu practitioners use the same channels and points as acupuncturists, but the points are called *tsubo* (*tsue-bo*). The term "shiatsu" came into being about 70 years ago to distinguish the use of fingers, thumbs, and palms as an actual medical treatment, instead of only for pleasure or relaxation.

Since then, shiatsu has become popular due to its simple and effective techniques. There are three legal manipulative therapies in Japan: *anma* (Japanese massage), western massage, and shiatsu. Shiatsu practitioners often use effective stretching techniques as well as pressure to unblock Qi channels and stimulate unrestricted flow. Shiatsu is often practiced on traditional soft cotton mats called futons. Your therapist will apply the steady and gentle pressure described throughout this book. Shiatsu often distinguishes itself from other forms of acupressure by involving Oriental Medical theory discussed in Chapter 6, and adopting many of the diagnostic procedures discussed in Chapter 2.

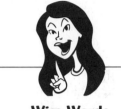

Wise Words

There is a tradition in Japan of blind shiatsu therapists. They are trained to greatly increase the sensitivity and skills of perception in their hands to give remarkable treatments.

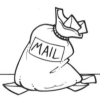

Mailbag

Brian was the manager of the engineering department at a local hotel. His job entailed both physical and mental labor. By the end of the week he was wiped out in both areas. Although he was unfamiliar with shiatsu or the concept of acupressure, he quickly let his apprehension go as he relaxed into a gentle yet rejuvenating treatment. Brian had thick, tight muscles that released into supple sinews following shiatsu's use of acu-points, channels, and stretching. At first he would make an appointment when he was wearing his shoulders like earrings, all hunched up and tight. Eventually, he discovered that with more regular treatments, he could feel well throughout his workweek and with his family.

Reflexology: Foot Geology

From ancient texts, illustrations, and artifacts, we know that the early Chinese, Japanese, Russians, Indians, and Egyptians applied pressure to different areas of the feet to promote good health. Today, many of these same techniques have been developed into a scientific method called reflexology. There are zones of energy that run throughout the body as well as reflex areas that correspond to all the major organs, glands, and body parts. Although many parts of the body such as the ears, hands, and scalp share this pattern, we will be focusing on the feet.

In the 1930s, Eunice Ingham, a physiotherapist, concluded that since the zones ran throughout the body and could be accessed anywhere, some areas might be more responsive than others. She was right: The feet were the most sensitive. She mapped out the entire body onto the feet. This map has been used universally ever since, with minor variations. Modern reflexology is an art and a science requiring study, practice, and skill. Since all the acupressure in reflexology is done on your feet, it is extremely safe and often indicated in conditions where the body can't be accessed at other locations, such as with certain types of cancer or a traumatic injury. Although your feet may find comfort by soaking in a warm tub of water or herbal solution, which will relax and soften the muscles, I find reflexology relaxes my whole body and begins the process of letting go of tension and stress. In reflexology, your feet may get the workout, but your whole body will reap the benefits.

Reflexology: Pressing on specific foot points can bring relief to your entire body.

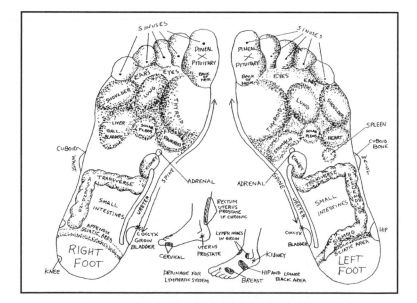

Types of Acupuncture: More Pointy Choices

You must be getting the point (no pun intended) that there are numerous healing systems from the Orient that developed over the centuries. Acupuncture styles, theories, and practices are as varied as the cultures they were perfected in.

Traditional Chinese Medicine (TCM)

Traditional Chinese medicine follows the 3,000-year-old principles of balancing the yin and yang of your body with its environment. These practitioners incorporate the science of all the natural forces that were observed and experienced by early healers (see Chapter 6, "How You Get Sick—The Good, the Bad, and the Ugly"). Practitioners make diagnoses using the techniques covered in Chapter 2, "What to Expect on Your First Visit—Does It Hurt?" and a wide variety of other techniques are applied to keep you feeling fit. Like Goldilocks, you want your energy "just right," for optimal health.

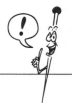

Acu-Moment

The Bronze Man was an early tool to learn acupuncture points. The figure was made of bronze and had 361 holes plugged with wax to represent the location of acu-points. The man was filled with water and dressed. The student was asked to find a point and insert a needle. If the location was wrong, the needle hit metal, but if it was correct, water spurted out. Glad that doesn't happen during a real treatment!

The history of TCM is filled with marvelous stories that illustrate a long search for understanding and teaching of medicine. One such tradition of which we have evidence is the famous Bronze Man, an instrument used in Traditional Chinese Medicine. The Bronze Man is actually made of bronze, the chief metal of the times and was used as a training tool for students learning to find acupoints. Many of these teaching and training techniques have been incorporated but using different materials. Most acupuncturists have a acu-man or acu-women in their office, but they're made of soft plastic instead of metal.

The Five-Element Tradition: Wooden You Like to Know

Since 400 B.C.E., the Chinese have understood their world through a distinct group of concepts: the five elements of wood, fire, earth, metal, and water.

These elements relate not only to symptoms that you are feeling, which a trained practitioner can categorize by color, odors, sounds, etc., but also how your body changes according to the relationships of the elements. Diagnosis is done through similar methods as described in TCM, with an added twist of arranging information to indicate a particular imbalance in an element and how that might affect the other elements, channels, or organs. Acupuncture treatment is given to specific points along the channels that correspond to elements that will help you regain balance and better health.

TABLE OF CORRESPONDENCES ASSOCIATED WITH THE FIVE PHASES					
	WOOD	FIRE	EARTH	METAL	WATER
Direction	East	South	Center	West	North
Season	Spring	Summer	Long Summer	Autumn	Winter
Climatic Condition	Wind	Summer Heat	Dampness	Dryness	Cold
Process	Birth	Growth	Transformation	Harvest	Storage
Color	Green	Red	Yellow	White	Black
Taste	Sour	Bitter	Sweet	Pungent	Salty
Smell	Goatish	Burning	Fragrant	Rank	Rotten
Yin Organ	Liver	Heart	Spleen	Lungs	Kidneys
Yang Organ	Gall Bladder	Small Intestine	Stomach	Large Intestine	Bladder
Opening	Eyes	Tongue	Mouth	Nose	Ears
Tissue	Sinews	Blood Vessels	Flesh	Skin/Hair	Bones
Emotion	Anger	Happiness	Pensiveness	Sadness	Fear
Human Sound	Shout	Laughter	Song	Weeping	Groan

Five elements at work in nature and you.

Japanese Acupuncture

The Japanese adapted many of the principles of Chinese medicine in order to develop their own style of diagnosis and treatment. Pulses are examined similarly as in TCM, but great emphasis is placed on the abdominal exam. The abdomen or *hara* (Sea of Qi) is believed to be the center of your body's energy, something like an energetic Times Square or Grand Central Station. From here, sensitive palpation can reveal a great deal about your system. Treatment is done through very shallow needle insertion, and the use of burning mugwort or moxa (see Chapter 5). TCM also uses moxa, but the practitioners of the Japanese style acupuncture have compiled and refined comprehensive treatments that balance your Qi, relieve symptoms, and promote health. Depending on your practitioner's style, you may also experience bio-magnetic acupuncture, which does not use any outside source of electricity, but calls on your body's own magnetic fields to adjust Qi flow.

It's an Acu-World After All

Over the last 3,000 years, Oriental Medicine has spread across our globe, fueled by increasing interest in finding ways to help us heal and balance our lives in our fast-paced world. As conventional "western" medicine merges with the time-tested principles of "eastern" medicine, the right combinations are being found to serve our world's need for effective healthcare. There are acupressure and acupuncture societies throughout the globe, and both are practiced in such countries as Germany, Israel, Ireland, Australia, Spain, Belgium, and Switzerland.

In the United States, 38 states and the District of Columbia have passed statutes or regulations for the practice of acupuncture with legislation pending in another 8 states. Forty acupuncture colleges in this country alone are accredited or in candidacy status. Acupuncture in many states is a three-year master's degree program, requiring a bachelor's degree with premed requirements. The healthful influences of these therapies are being felt worldwide.

Acu-points have gone global!

Now you've learned the roots of acupressure and acupuncture. The different styles of acupressure's shiatsu and reflexology and the multiple contributions of many countries such as China, Japan, England, and the United States have made Oriental Medicine a diverse healing system. In the next chapter, we're going right into the therapeutic techniques of acupressure with what to do and how to do it. Grab a partner and your favorite futon and get ready to practice.

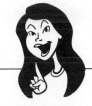

Wise Words

General Douglas MacArthur banned all Oriental Medicine in Japan after WWII because he thought it unscientific. The Japanese Blind Shiatsu Association contacted Helen Keller, who wrote President Harry Truman and convinced him to change the law. In Tokyo, there is a shiatsu and acupuncture school mainly for the blind named after Helen Keller.

The Least You Need to Know

➤ Oriental Medicine dates back over 3,000 years.

➤ Chinese medicine began as separate traditions in the northern and southern parts of the country, later merging into one system.

➤ The Japanese term *shiatsu* means "finger" (*shi*) "pressure" (*atsu*).

➤ The Five Elements can help a traditional Oriental diagnostician develop a diagnosis and treatment plan.

➤ There are over 40 acupuncture colleges in the United States.

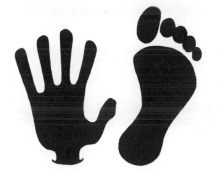

Chapter 4

Acupressure— Fingers, Hands, and a Whole Lot More

In This Chapter

➤ Learn how to use your fingers, palms, and feet to release tired and sore muscles

➤ Know how hard to push before you go too far

➤ Discover the three kinds of pressure and when to use them

➤ Activate your Qi channels with these stimulating, easy-to-learn techniques

---

I used to hear the same excuses from my friends and family every time I wanted them to give me an acupressure treatment. "Oh, I can't do that …. I don't know how." This chapter is for all the people who would like to learn the simple yet powerful techniques used in acupressure or have an idea exactly how your acu-pro works.

By reading this chapter and following the pictures, you'll feel more confident in the way you perform acupressure, including just the right amount of pressure. Every time you practice, your sensitivity will increase. By asking yourself and others how they feel afterward, you'll continue to guide yourself along in the right direction of healing and centered relaxation. So, no more excuses: It's time to give the best acupressure session there is. Let's go for it!

From Fingers to Feet—Using Your Body to Heal

When performing acupressure either on yourself or others, think about what you want to accomplish; do you want to help someone relax a sore muscle, increase circulation, or improve his or her digestion? In Oriental Medical traditions in addition to just knowing which points to use, thinking about your intended result helps focus your mind and center your own healing potential. No matter which technique or breathing pattern you use, remember to bring along my two favorite companions: heart and soul!

Fingers and Palms ... Hold On!

Palm pressure is noted for its soothing penetration to acu-points and larger muscle groups. Your palm and finger should be relaxed, letting the natural shape and contour of the muscle determine the exact hand position (see the following figure).

Your thumb is an important tool to press on acu-points, but it's not big enough to carry the entire burden of the treatment. Use your fingers to support and protect the workhorse of the hand—your thumb.

Your elbow is used to stimulate acu-points that are located in deep layers of muscle or fatty tissue that can't be reached by your fingers or thumb. I also use my elbows to break up stubborn muscle knots that have resisted more gentle approaches. By using proper body alignment and balance, firm yet comfortable pressure can be applied through your elbow that might otherwise quickly fatigue your palms or fingers.

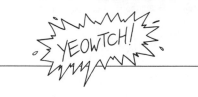

Harm Alarm

Don't tire yourself out! Pressing on acu-points can be hard work. Use fingers to reinforce and support your thumb. Spread out the workload so you can keep on pressing like a pro.

Relaxed palm and fingers conform to the shape of the muscle and can deliver consistent pressure.

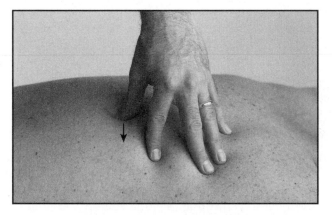

Support your thumb with a relaxed fist, which rests flat against the skin

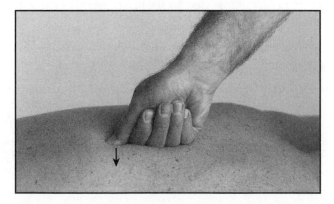

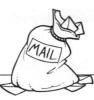

Mailbag

Stacey worked on her feet in a grocery store all day long. By midday she felt a tightening of her hips and buttocks area that would spasm frequently during the afternoon, which made it challenging for her to work the whole day and even more difficult for her to funtion later that night as a single parent of two children. I diagnosed her condition as a stuck or stagnant Qi in the channels from overuse, resulting in tight, sore muscles. When I applied direct vertical pressure to her hips she felt sore while I was pressing, while experiencing a great sense of pain relief following the techniques. I used a combination of vertical pressure with my elbow in which I could control the application of sustained direct pressure, and stretching. As she improved, I taught her how to do the acupressure with a tennis ball and continue with the streching on her own. The last time I was in the store she was beaming with a smile.

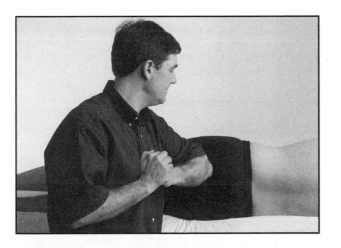

Your elbow is a great tool for deep or stubborn muscle knots. Staying balanced and aligned will help you deliver firm yet gentle relief.

Feet: Please Tread on Me

Believe it or not, having your back walked on can be one of the most relaxing acupressure techniques you'll ever experience. Let me explain that only thoroughly qualified, petite practitioners get to walk on the muscles on either side of your spine—and never directly on it! They have been specially trained to feel your tense muscles with sensitivity in their feet, much like you may have in your hands. They let their weight (which isn't much) sink slowly and carefully into your back.

*Feet are an effective tool
for firm, contoured
pressure.*

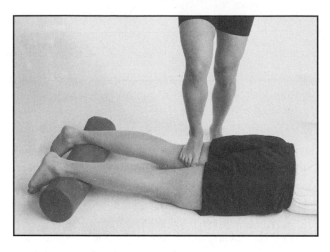

Most of the time, feet are used to press acu-points much like you would use the palm. One foot is on the floor while the other delivers contoured pressure over a larger muscle area such as the back, arms, or legs. I would suggest only doing work on the back if you've had specific training.

Pressure on the Point—How Hard Do You Push?

Acupressure uses firm yet gentle penetrating pressure on acu-points. These points may already be sore to the touch, so go easy. Healing is not a horse race. Keep asking your subject if the pressure feels good, or if it is so strong that it keeps you or your subject from relaxing.

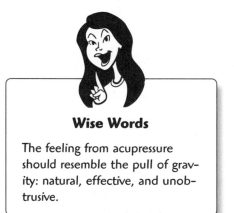

Wise Words

The feeling from acupressure should resemble the pull of gravity: natural, effective, and unobtrusive.

Many acupressure therapists develop abilities to sense the Qi in the acu-points. The books and charts will get you close to the right acu-point, sensing will put you on the mark. I locate points by going to the general area and then wait to feel the energy of the point. Sometimes it's a warm or tingling feeling, or a small buzz or spark. Other times I feel the energy sink in or push back against me. In my experience, sensing the energy of the point, either drawing you in (deficient Qi) or pushing you away (excessive Qi), is part of the real art and skill of acupressure.

Three Types of Pressure

The first question most of my patients interested in acupressure ask me is "How hard do I push?" The amount or type of pressure is determined by the condition. A simple test is to press gently into an area that hurts. Does that feel better or worse with firm direct pressure? If a condition feels worse with pressure, it usually means that there is not enough Qi or Qi circulation in the area. You'll read more about this condition in

Chapter 6, "How You Get Sick—The Good, the Bad, and the Ugly." In such cases, you'll want to apply more gentle and stationary pressure. Firmer more vertical pressure aids areas that have too much Qi stuck in them and feel relieved following this more direct pressure.

➤ **Vertical.** Pressing straight into the skin for three to five seconds.

➤ **Stationary.** Applying pressure while holding an acu-point or points. Holding points for 2–30 seconds can help open energy channels, relax muscles, and calm internal organs.

➤ **Supporting.** Allowing your own Qi to support the healing of another. Sometimes the mental focus or intention you have will dissolve the blockage better than physical pressure alone.

I recommend that you keep your mind focused on your desired intentional outcome—support for all of the acupressure techniques used. Combining your mental and physical energies is essential to giving a successful acupressure treatment.

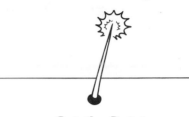

Get the Point

The strength, stability, and power of acupressure come from the ability to move your body's weight evenly through your elbows, into your fingers. Rikyu, founder and master of the Japanese Tea Ceremony, once said, "Don't shake your tea whisk with your fingertips, but with your elbow."

Common Acupressure Techniques— Shake, Rattle, and Roll

This is where the rubber hits the road. It's time to practice a few of the acupressure techniques on a friend or family member. Remember to be gentle and read carefully before starting. These techniques are safe and easy to perform with a little practice, so lay the book beside you and have fun learning acupressure.

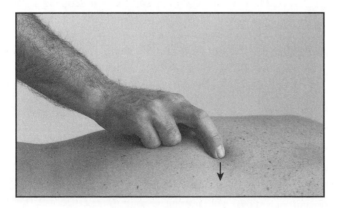

Your index finger is bent to support the thumb. Apply firm vertical pressure with thumb and index finger.

Lightly pinch and pull up muscles before applying thumb or palm pressure.

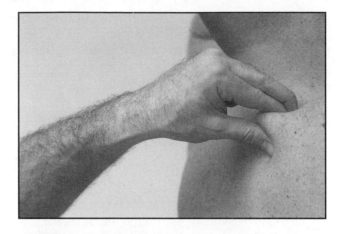

Place one palm on the top, forming crossed hands, for more controlled and even pressure.

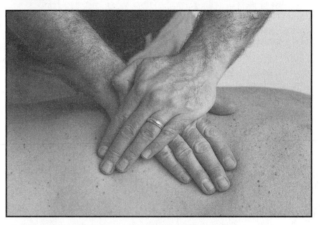

Tapping increases circulation and invigorates tired muscles. Lightly tap with palms or fingertips. Relax your fingers, moving your wrists and elbows. I recommend tapping lightly for 5–15 seconds on a point to loosen tight, congested Qi. A little tap will do ya!

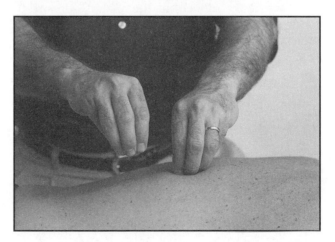

I hope you have gained some understanding of the considerable training that an acupressure therapist goes through in order to get the ooooos and aaaahs from you. With practice you can be quite the popular one in your house. Next we'll move onto acupuncture, which I'd leave up to the pros. Would you be surprised to learn that needles are only a portion of what they've got to help you with? Read on!

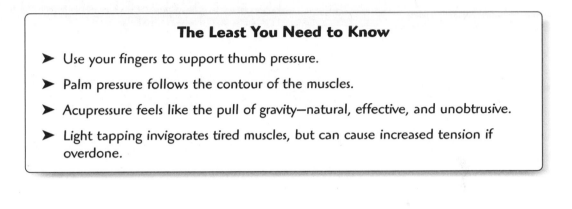

The Least You Need to Know

➤ Use your fingers to support thumb pressure.

➤ Palm pressure follows the contour of the muscles.

➤ Acupressure feels like the pull of gravity—natural, effective, and unobtrusive.

➤ Light tapping invigorates tired muscles, but can cause increased tension if overdone.

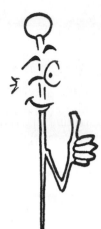

Chapter 5

Acupuncture— Tools of the Trade

In This Chapter

➤ Know what other tools acupuncturists have in their bags to help you

➤ Discover how to eat with the seasons using oriental methods of nutrition

➤ Are medicinal herbs right for you?

Patients of mine are usually surprised by the different types of treatments available to them. I completely understand. When you go to see an acupuncturist, you would think all it would involve is a few needles here and there. Not necessarily so. Acupuncturists today have a vast array of tools in their goodie bags ready to be tailored to fit your exact condition.

In this chapter, you'll discover what acupuncture needles look like, and why they don't hurt. We'll discuss the progression of acupuncture healing tools, from chunky pieces of stone to a modern, hair-like, surgical stainless steel disposable needles. You'll learn about the therapeutic benefits of a hollowed-out horn of an animal ... a method accomplished today without the horn from the animal! Many of the techniques covered in this chapter can also be a bridge to your own self-care. Learning them can get you feeling better and stronger with the effects lasting longer. So keep reading!

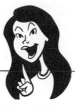

Wise Words

No pain and lots of gain are what you get from modern acupuncture. When you think of needles, I'll bet you think of the shot in the arm you get from your doctor. Hypodermic needles are chisel-shaped to cut through muscles and large enough to inject medicine. Acupuncture needles are small and hairlike, carrying no medicine in or on the needle. They have rounded tips to slide through muscle, not cut it. That's why they don't hurt!

Needles: When Size Does Matter

Acupuncture uses needles inserted beneath the superficial layer of the skin to simulate the underlying points and channels to correct and maintain good health. The idea is to keep your Qi, your life energy, flowing smoothly through your body. Pain is said to be "stuck Qi." Acupuncture needles move the Qi along its pathways ... head 'em up, and move 'em out.

The earliest acupuncture needles were made of stone (remember the Flintstones?). They were called *bian*, which is a Chinese term that means "using stone to treat disease." As tools and technology changed, so did the needles. The quest for the best needle continued from bone to bamboo, through ceramic, bronze, and iron, then to steel. Several gold and silver acupuncture needles were discovered in a 2,000-year-old tomb in Hebei province, proving you *can* take it with you. Today, most needles are very fine and made from stainless steel, although some practitioners use silver, gold, copper, or zinc needles for their electrical conductivity properties.

Acupuncture needles are thin, hair-like, and painless. After all, comfort counts!

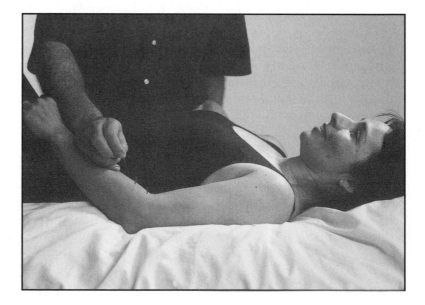

Needle Knowledge

In 1996, the U.S. Food and Drug Administration approved the use of acupuncture needles as medical devices. The acupuncture needles are made of high-quality surgical stainless steel that are so thin they might remind you of a strand of hair. Although most practitioners use sterile disposable needles, your practitioner will give you a choice of either sterilized, reusable needles or disposable needles thrown out after each use.

Students of acupuncture practice using these needles on pieces of fruit or tightly bound foam to acquire just the right skill. Inserted quickly and gently, acupuncture patients feel nothing but a slight pinch. When you arrive at your first acupuncture appointment, your acu-pro will choose needles of lengths and sizes appropriate for your body type and condition. The practitioner may put in and take out a needle quickly, or may have you relax while the needle stays put for about 20 to 30 minutes in order to move Qi blocked within the acu-point. The practitioner may decide to add mild electrical stimulation to aid in greater Qi movement.

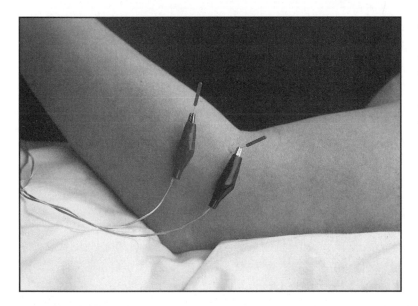

A mild electric current may be connected to the acupuncture needles to enhance the circulation. This technique is frequently used in cases of severe or chronic pain and dysfunction.

Electromagnetic acupuncture.

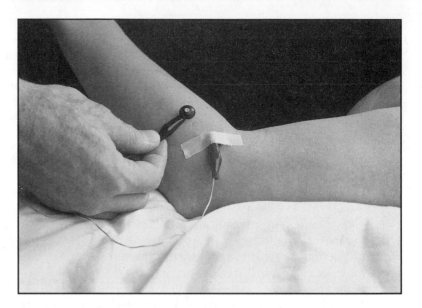

Electromagnetic acupuncture is a non-needle technique, using magnets that have a mild electrical current that passes through the magnet and stimulates the acu-points and channels. You may feel a light tapping or a little buzzy sensation on your skin. I use this technique frequently for joint pain and injuries or where the area may be too sensitive to the patient for needle acupuncture.

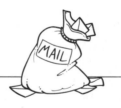

Mailbag

Al is a truck driver for a large national company and typically puts in a 70-hour work-week. While he was out on his snowmobile, he felt his right ankle begin to ache. By the time he went to bed his right ankle was swollen, and by the next day it was difficult for him to put much weight on it without a lot of pain. He tried driving, but had to cut back and finally stop driving due to his pain. His diagnosis from his physician was an ankle sprain, but meds and physical therapy had not helped him so far. I used a combination of needle and electromagnetic acupuncture to reduce his swelling and ease the pain. Following the first treatment, the swelling had reduced considerably, and during the next three weeks I used Tui-Na massage and external herbal wraps and finally taught him home exercises and bio-magnetic treatments to do daily. His progress was consistent and he can manage any daily discomfort from overwork with his home treatments.

Moxibustion—A Real Warm-Up

Moxibustion is a technique that uses *moxa* (mugwort or *Artemisia vulgaris*) burned on or above the skin to warm acu-points and channels using the dried, wool-like leaves of this plant. It's no surprise that Stone Age cave dwellers who lived in damp, cold conditions felt better when they were warmed in this way. The Chinese created effective ways to heal faster by having a live coal or burning stick either touching the skin or warming the acu-points. Moxa was such an important part of acupuncture that the Chinese name for acupuncture, *Zhen Jiu*, means needle and burning.

Today moxibustion is used for any condition that is worse from cold or that benefits from the penetrating heat of this smoldering plant, such as abdominal pain, diarrhea, arthritis, and gynecological disorders. Moxibustion is safe and effective when performed by a trained professional. The leaves are picked in the spring when they're fresh and dried. They are then ground into a fine powder, filtered to remove any dirt or coarse materials, and washed and dried several times until the wool-like material can be molded in cones or sticks.

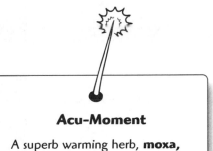

Acu-Moment

A superb warming herb, **moxa,** also called mugwort or *Artemisia vulgaris,* is a plant that grows in China and even throughout North America. The leaves are powdered, washed, and dried to form a wool-like material that can be shaped into sticks or cones.

Moxibustion: The Cherry on Top

As mentioned previously, moxibustion uses the plant mugwort or *Artemisia vulgaris*, which herbalists have scraped, washed, and left to dry for a full three to seven years. If you touched the mugwort before your practitioner burned it, it would feel like soft woolen fibers that have been molded into sticks or cones.

Your acu-pro can use moxibustion in two ways. He or she can place it directly on your skin, either by itself or with a paste made from ginger, garlic, salt, or pepper. The other method is more indirect: The acu-pro lights a stick of moxa and holds it over the acu-point the heat is meant to affect. The heat from the burning plant warms the channels and increases circulation of Qi, especially if your condition is worse from cold. Your practitioner's style and training will probably determine whether he or she decides to use direct or indirect moxibustion.

There are some times when you shouldn't use moxibustion, including the following:

➤ Do not use moxibustion if you have a fever.

➤ Do not use moxibustion on the low back or abdomen of pregnant women.

➤ Do not use direct moxibustion on the face or other sensory organs, in the breast area, or over large blood vessels or tendons.

Today, practitioners can use an infrared heat lamp instead of moxa, and they often use hot or cold packs in the office and as take-home self-care therapies.

Moxa on a stick—a convenient, commercially prepared way to warm acu-points.

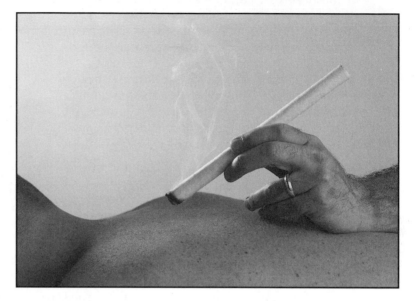

Cupping: Trying to Horn In

An animal horn was hollowed out and placed over infected tissue to drain out old blood and puss. Yuck! Putting heat near the opening created the suction for the horns and a vacuum that pulled the skin and goo into the horn. This did work, however, and soon bamboo, ceramic, brass, and iron containers that looked liked cups were being used. (You'll never use a cup the same way again, will you?)

Despite how it sounds, it's very weird and wonderful all at the same time. Today cupping is used for a wide variety of conditions (for example, arthritis, headache, low-back pain, painful menstruation, and the common cold). The gentle pulling of your skin into the cup is a little like a hug from an octopus, except you don't get wet and it's better for you.

Cupping Comments

Today, cups are made of glass and come in a variety of sizes to fit specific body surfaces. Some models have a suction pump to pull out the air and create a vacuum, while other models use heat to create the same effect. A practitioner may place either a single cup or multiple cups on acu-points to break up stuck Qi and relieve pain. Again, this process shouldn't be painful, but your skin can be temporarily reddened, raised, and have a bruised look following treatment, but it won't be sore.

Here are several different ways that practitioners use cupping:

➤ Cup edges can be lubricated and placed over large, flat areas of the back or legs, and then moved up and down to strongly increase Qi flow.

➤ Cups can be put over needles that are placed in acu-points for deeper stimulation.

➤ Cups can be placed on your body while containing different herbs such as ginger juice or hot pepper water.

Your practitioner will not use cupping to treat fever, convulsions, allergic skin conditions, or ulcerated sores.

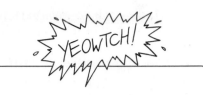

Harm Alarm

Your acupuncturist should not attempt to place cups on angular body areas or place them too close together. This will cause unnecessary discomfort when pulling the surrounding skin too tightly.

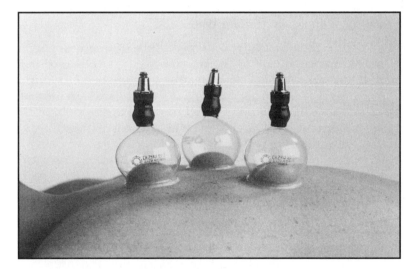

Cupping unknots the sore muscles of your back.

Massage and Exercise: Movin', Movin', Movin'

You've probably figured out by now that keeping your Qi moving plays a big part in healing illnesses and staying healthy. Oriental Medicine incorporates massage (Tui-Na) and numerous exercises (medical Qi Gong) into the training of health professionals.

Tui-Na: Push Me, Pull You

This oriental massage technique, safe for both children and adults, uses pressing, rubbing, kneading, and pinching to bring your body back into balance. In fact, *Tui-Na* means "push" *(too-ee)* and "grasp" *(nah)*. The practitioner massages acu-points and energy channels to promote healthy Qi flow and organ function, and Traditional Chinese Medicine hospitals have Tui-Na departments along with acupuncture wards for combined healthcare.

As is true for most other methods, Tui-Na isn't for everyone. Practitioners will avoid using Tui-Na on

➤ A pregnant woman's abdomen, low back, or other contraindicated acu-points (see Chapter 16, "Birthing Baby").

➤ Tumors (see Chapter 15, "Cancer—A Ray of Hope").

Medical Qi Gong—It's a Bird, It's a Crane, It's You!

Another way to improve your health is through the practice of medical *Qi Gong*. Qi ("life energy") and *gong* ("benefits from persistent efforts") are combined with slow, easy-to-perform breathing exercises to assist a wide variety of health concerns. Medical Qi Gong can be prescribed by your acu-pro for helping specific conditions such as cancer, arthritis, and many muscular or joint pains.

Qi Gong helps to circulate Qi through channels by easy-to-perform slow movements (which often mimic the movements of animals the originators may have observed in nature) such as the tiger, deer, crane, or monkey) and breathing techniques. Qi Gong is very versatile, and people of every age and in any physical condition can find poses that will work for them, since Qi Gong can be practiced while standing up, seated, or lying down.

Two types of Qi Gong include

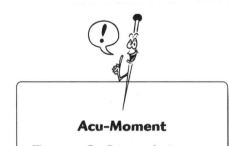

Acu-Moment

The term **Qi Gong** is fairly recent, first used in 1936 in Dong Hao's work, *Special Therapy for Tuberculosis*. Today it has come to mean all of the therapeutic breathing exercises from the Shaman animal dances of the Zhou Dynasty (1028–221 B.C.E.) to the popular slow motion early morning routines practiced by millions of Chinese in open-air parks.

➤ **Wei Dan.** Moves your body's Qi through physical activity such as moving your arms or walking. Many beginners start off with this method because its movements create the Qi flow. You can add more advanced breathing and visualizations once you learn the sequence and your mind is calmer.

➤ **Nei Dan.** Moves your body's Qi through mental activity and imagery alone. This form can be as simple as breathing in and out while remembering a peaceful moment, or a highly intricate system of breathing techniques and sensing that enables you to circulate your Qi through every channel and organ in your body.

If you're using Qi Gong, let your conventional physician know because Qi Gong training can affect the dosage requirements of insulin, chemotherapy, or medications for high blood pressure.

Magnets: What's the Attraction?

Pick up any magazine these days and you'll notice that many ads on the back pages involve the use of magnets. However popular magnets may be today, the use of magnets as medical tools is not a new fad. In fact, civilizations such as China, India, and Egypt used magnets to treat ailments for centuries, and today magnetic therapy has officially been accepted as a medical procedure in Germany, Japan, Israel, Russia, and 45 other countries.

In Oriental Medicine, magnets are used to set up specific patterns of flow, using the bioelectrical and magnetic properties of Qi. Although no one completely understands how they work, practitioners use magnets to treat such conditions as arthritis, back pain, bursitis, carpal tunnel, and tennis elbow.

Before using therapeutic magnets, check with your acu-pro or family physician to avoid buying an ineffective product or risk an unknown contraindication with other therapies or devices you're using.

Nutrition: Heal with the Energy of Food

Oriental Medicine recognizes how important food and nutrition are to our health. Sun Shu Mao in 652 C.E. wrote a book, *One Thousand Ounces of Gold Classic;* no, he didn't charge that much to buy it, but he did believe that human life and health was worth that much. His book detailed acupuncture, herbal, and dietary treatments for various common ailments of the times.

Your acu-pro may have studied complementary nutrition and can assist you in choosing supplements to complement your care. He or she may have also studied the oriental system of food therapy. Foods, like herbs, have been traditionally categorized by the energy they have (food Qi) and the reactions they cause once you've eaten them. Food therapy owes much of its logic to Chinese herbal

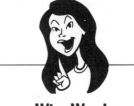

Wise Words

Lodestones are natural magnetic rocks used by early sailors for navigation purposes (lodestar or leading star). Queen Cleopatra of Egypt was rumored to have worn a lodestone on her forehead while she slept to prevent wrinkles and aging.

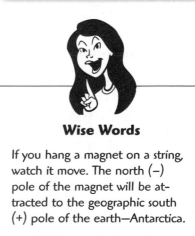

Wise Words

If you hang a magnet on a string, watch it move. The north (−) pole of the magnet will be attracted to the geographic south (+) pole of the earth—Antarctica.

45

medicine. Specific foods can be recommended based on your condition and underlying health. Your food becomes an important part of self-care.

The Healing Power of Food

Foods have five flavors that affect your internal organs:

➤ Pungent (acidic)—Lungs and large intestine

➤ Sweet—Stomach and spleen

➤ Sour—Liver and gallbladder

➤ Bitter—Heart and small intestine

➤ Salty—Kidney and bladder

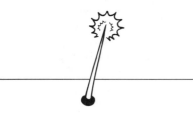

Get the Point

Take ginger for a cold! Fresh grated ginger or ginger juice may be added to soup one minute before it's removed from the stove. Ginger increases the warmth in your body and traditionally is thought to increase circulation in the outer muscles of the head and upper back, driving the cold out.

Flavors have specific action on the organs:

➤ Pungent (acidic) (ginger, peppermint)— Promotes circulation and perspiration

➤ Sweet (honey, sugar, watermelon)—Slows down acute symptoms and improves digestion

➤ Sour (lemons, plums)—Slows down excessive diarrhea or perspiration

➤ Bitter (coffee, hops, vinegar)—Reduces body heat or fevers and dry body fluids, or induces diarrhea

➤ Salty (barley, crab, seaweed)—Softens hard nodules like goiter

The five energies of food are described by what the foods do in our bodies. Once you eat them, do you feel hot, cold, warm, cool, or neutral? Foods also tend to affect specific areas of the body: When you eat certain foods, do you feel sensations inside or on the surface of your body? In your upper or lower body?

You can also alter food energies depending on how you prepare them. Pan frying (without oil) toasts the outside of the food and develops a warming effect felt in the lower part of your body, which means that food prepared that way can help alleviate low-back pain or certain menstrual irregularities.

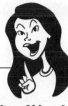

Herbal Medicine—Plants Plus

Medicinal herbs have become increasingly popular in our culture. It seems that most new supplements or power bars have some unusual-sounding Chinese herb as an ingredient. Magazine covers announce herbs to aid you in a wide variety of complaints.

It is thought that humans learned which herbs were safe to eat from animals. Animals have an intuitive sense of which herbs to eat when they are sick, while we had to experiment through trial and error.

Oriental herbal medicine is a complete system of diagnosis (see Chapter 2, "What to Expect on Your First Visit—Does It Hurt?") and treatments, using plants, minerals, and traditionally some animals and insects (chocolate-covered cricket, anyone?). Herbal traditions come from many countries such as China, Korea, and Japan, but we typically roll them all together and call it Chinese herbal medicine. Oriental herbalists learn techniques for combining many herbs in a single formula to help you with complex medical conditions. For instance, herbs used to treat fibromyalgia (see Chapter 7, "Pain from the Neck Up") reduce pain and also increase your energy and stamina.

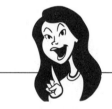

The practice of herbal medicine declined in this country with the new use of sulfa drugs and antibiotics. Herbal practices are making a comeback with patients who want a whole-health approach to wellness that is not as disease-focused as conventional medicine.

At your first herbal consult, your acu-pro will review your specific concerns and your overall health. When the imbalances in your system have been identified, a custom prescription in pill, powder, etc., will be ordered or given to you in the office. Your herbalist may also give you pre-made herbal products.

Make sure you understand the instructions for taking your herbs, how much they will cost new, and approximately how often they need to be refilled. Ask the source of these herbs and avoid any illegal ingredients such as endangered animals like rhino horn or tiger bones. They are rarely used in the United States and more common overseas where demand unfortunately still persists. Typically, you'll schedule follow-up visits to check on your progress about every month at first and then at longer intervals as your condition improves. One of the advantages of a custom-made prescription is that all substances can be changed or substituted in order to find the best formula for you.

Here are a few tips to get you started:

➤ Herbs help balance your body. For example, if you are cold, your practitioner will prescribe herbs that will warm you.

➤ Herbs are categorized into the five temperatures that you feel from taking them: hot, cold, warm, cool, and neutral.

➤ The five tastes or effects herbs have on your body's organs are acidic, sweet, bitter, sour, and salty.

You'll find that herbs come in several different forms, each with its own advantages and disadvantages. These forms include

➤ **Pills (*wan*).** Powdered herbs are mixed with an edible thick substance, then to rolled together to form hard pills.

➤ **Decoctions (*tang ji*).** Raw herbs are placed in water or a mixture of wine and water and then boiled. The liquid is strained off and drunk as a tea that is rapidly absorbed in the body.

➤ **Powders (*san*).** Many people prefer to use herbs in powdered form because they are more readily absorbed by the body and are easy to store.

➤ **Syrups (*gao*).** Herbs are boiled till thick and concentrated, then sugar or honey is added. Many prescriptions that use honey therapeutically such as cough syrups rely on this tasty and convenient way to take herbs.

➤ **Plasters (*gao yao*).** In order to form plasters, powdered herbs are added to a heated mixture of oil, put on cloth, and applied externally to skin problems or painful muscles or joints.

➤ **Medicinal wines (*jiu*).** Medicinal herbs are sometimes steeped in wine (this is one wine you won't find in Napa Valley!).

I told you there were a lot of choices when it came to acupuncturist's tools. We've seen how they can use hair-like needles alone, with electricity, or even be replaced by several non-needle techniques such as electromagnetic acupuncture. Warming with moxa, clearing soreness or opening lungs with cupping, massage, oriental nutrition, or herbs can be used by your acupuncturist to serve your needs.

In the next chapter, we'll explore the factors that influence health. You'll find out the difference between the wind that messes up your hair and the Wind that gives you a headache!

The Least You Need to Know

➤ Acupuncture needles don't hurt, because they are hair-thin and round-tipped to glide between muscle fibers.

➤ Moxibustion increases circulation by heating up acu-points with the controlled burning of herbs.

➤ Cupping pulls and lifts muscles into a glass jar to untie the knots.

➤ Acu-pros can teach you about medicinal foods and exercises to keep you feeling good long after your treatment has ended.

➤ Chinese herbal medicines are customized to your exact needs and change as your condition improves.

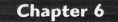

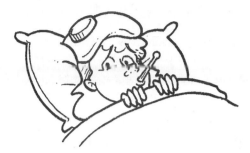

Chapter 6

How You Get Sick—The Good, the Bad, and the Ugly

In This Chapter

➤ What are yin and yang, and what do they have to do with your health

➤ Find out the source of your energy

➤ Learn how you can be under the weather ... literally

How in the world does your acu-pro know what's going on with you? In this chapter, we'll take a look at how your acu-pro breaks down all the things you say into patterns that have been bothering people for thousands of years.

These patterns could be signs of health and well-being that show a history of resistance to illness, or they could point to gaps in your armor and susceptibility to disease. Do you feel like you'll get sick on a cold, damp day? This chapter will explain patterns that Oriental Medical practitioners have been observing for over 2,000 years. This form of medicine puts a lot of focus on prevention and early treatment. Let's fact it, your health is like a balancing weight scale; if the strength of the disease on one side is bigger and badder than you are, then sickness results. Your acu-pro's job is to understand the patterns in your health and help you balance the scales in your favor.

Yin and Yang—the Great Balancing Act

Perhaps the best recognized symbol of oriental philosophy is the Yin and Yang sign called *taiji* or the Great Polarity. From old cowboy movies, we often mistakenly attach the meaning of good to the white side and bad to the black side. Actually, no such judgment is meant in this sign. The symbol shows how it takes both opposites to complement one another in perfect harmony. This is the broadest definition of balance in Oriental Medicine.

The earliest reference to Yin and Yang is probably in the "Book of Changes" written by Yi Jing at about 700 B.C.E. The Yin-Yang school of philosophy developed, as many other philosophies did, during the Warring States period in China (476-221 B.C.E.) As the name suggests, China was embroiled in war, lives were turned upside down, and schools of philosophy developed in an attempt to make sense of it all. Yin and Yang is as simple as it is profound. I have listed the simple correspondences that Chinese farmers observed in nature along with a couple of medical comparisons in a table below.

Both my Oriental Medical training and martial arts have taught me that the nature of Yin and Yang is more dynamic than a static chart. Take another look at the *taiji* symbol. Notice the small seed or dot of white inside the black color and visa versa. This shows us that nothing is totally Yin or Yang and that all things including humans have the ability to change and transform. The symbol further illustrates this by its shape. Think of the symbol moving in a clockwise direction (although it can be reversed). As the white color is at its peak of growth and expansion the dark color begins to take over gradually until it too diminishes continuing the never-ending cycle in nature and in our bodies. We all carry within us the necessary energies to balance and heal. Often I find it useful to search for the hidden seed of transformation within a condition or situation.

The Yin and Yang sign illustrates the ability to achieve balance in an ever-changing world.

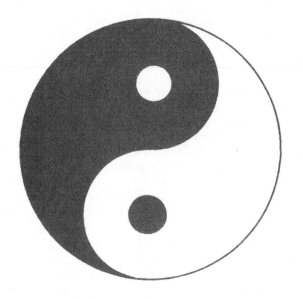

Yin	Yang
Female	Male
Night	Day

Inside	Outside
Front	Back
Lower Body	Upper Body
Bones	Skin
Blood	Qi
Too Little	Too Much

Qi and Blood: Building Blocks of Health

We've talked about qi before as the life's energy that circulates throughout the body. The word "blood" to western minds is the red stuff in our veins. In Oriental Medicine, think of it as having a more dynamic job of traveling side-by-side with Qi to nourish all parts of your body. They are the tag team of health protection in your system.

Qi in Oriental Medical terms means the energy of life. We receive Qi when we are born and continue to be given Qi through many sources including the air we breathe and the food we eat. Our bodies use Qi to accomplish daily living and each organ and channel is filled with this life energy to assist with the simplest or complex tasks.

Your acu-pro may be treating your Stomach Qi for poor digestion or your Lung Qi when you have a cough or asthma. These are examples of the functional aspect of Qi for organs. Qi also circulates throughout your body helping to nourish it with necessary blood and fluids. Remember that Qi is the unseen energy that supports your body's known and visible functions. The strength of your Qi will manifest in your physical, mental, and emotional states. This is why your acu-pro will want to know about all of these areas.

Blood has an additional meaning in Oriental Medicine than what most of us grew up with. Blood is seen as a form of Qi that flows through our veins and carries the energy of Qi within to nourish and moisten your body. A common strategy in Oriental Medicine for dry skin is to eat foods and herbs that strengthen the blood aspect in your body. A relative deficiency in blood can also lead to mental restlessness, forgetfulness, or insomnia. These correspondences have been observed, treated, and explained by the concept of the energy that your blood possesses.

➤ **Deficient Qi.** Symptoms of a deficient Qi include fatigue, depression, pale complexion, or pale swollen tongue with teeth marks on the edges.

➤ **Stuck Qi.** If your Qi is "stuck," you're likely to feel a dull pain, bloating, or fullness in chest or abdomen.

➤ **Deficient blood.** A condition involving deficient blood may cause dizziness, pale complexion, dry skin, loss of hair, pale lips and tongue, and a thin pulse.

➤ **Stuck blood.** If your blood is "stuck," you'll probably feel a localized, fixed, stabbing pain.

The Dreaded Excesses: Too Much, Too Fast

According to traditional Oriental Medicine, there are six weather conditions that, if they come at you when you are weak or tired, can cause you to become sick. This explains why an acu-pro will treat two people with the flu or a cold in different ways, depending on how their bodies react to the outside environment.

Over a few thousand years, Oriental medical practitioners have observed that illnesses come about from either an external influence that you are susceptible to such as weather or environmental pollutants or internal weaknesses brought on by chronic sickness or poor lifestyle choices. External weather patterns that create illness in those that are in a weakened or susceptible state have been seen to be more prominent at certain times of the year. If you have a weakness, such as deficient digestive Qi, and are exposed to excessive dampness, either through the weather or poor diet, then you will take on some of the characteristics of dampness. Late summer has been the traditionally observed time of year when dampness has the most profound effect on those that are open to it. Take a look at these characters and see where your weaknesses may lie.

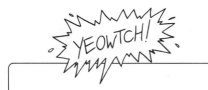

Harm Alarm

It's normal to have emotions, but if one emotion gets stuck and keeps going ... watch out! Traditionally, the seven emotions that can be too much for you are happiness, anger, worry, pensiveness, sadness, fear, and terror. Stuck emotions can lead to excessive behavior such as road rage or anxiety.

The Bothersome Barometer

Each pathogenic character in Oriental Medicine has a time of year that this aspect of illness is felt strongly in the environment. If you are at a weakened state of health or the influence is overwhelmingly strong, you will most likely develop some of the symptoms noted with each weather characteristic in the following list. If you observe each season, I believe you will consistently see for yourself the correspondences written and observed over thousands of years ago.

➤ **Wind (spring).** Illness comes on suddenly, changes quickly, or moves around. Includes spasms, itching, vertigo, moving pain.

➤ **Cold (winter).** You feel cold and your body contracts (sound familiar?). Cold causes pain from stuck Qi and blood.

➤ **Heat (no season).** Feels hot and can dry you out. Symptoms are fever, headache, rash, constipation, and dry cough, while mucus is dark or yellow, sticky, and foul-smelling.

➤ **Dampness (late summer).** Too much moisture or damp weather. Symptoms include feeling sluggish, heavy and swollen, numbness, and fixed dull pain.

➤ **Dryness (fall).** Dries up the moisture of your body (like a dry, crisp fall leaf); dry skin, chapped lips, dry hacking cough, and constipation.

➤ **Summer heat (summer).** Produces excessive sweating with very little or no physical exertion. Can't stop perspiring, even when it's not hot.

The Directions of Disease: Follow the Yellow Brick Road

How bad is it? That's one of the first questions on the minds of both the patient and the acu-pro at any given appointment. Oriental Medicine helps organize the possibilities by using the eight principles of any illness. These broad opposites give us a starting point for diagnosing the condition and determining how your body is dealing with it in general terms. As we discussed in Chapter 2, "What to Expect on Your First Visit—Does It Hurt?" the acu-pro refines this diagnosis and selects a treatment that's right for you.

The Eight Directions: Which Way Did He Go?

The identification of patterns according to the eight directions is the foundation for all other methods of diagnosis in Traditional Chinese Medicine (TCM). By looking at your condition, your acu-pro will determine the basic location and nature of the disharmony that has led to your illness.

The following descriptions are meant to be guidelines and are often mixed in an actual patient. It is not unusual for a patient to exhibit the external symptoms of a cold, while suffering from the internal discomfort of asthma. Now you may see why your acu-pro spends so much time in school. The true purpose of using the eight directions is not to make a person fit into a category, rather to foster an understanding of the origins and nature of an illness. Take a look at the following list. Which direction are you following?

➤ **Exterior/Interior.** Sore muscles or skin problems are exterior, while organ dysfunction is related to the interior.

➤ **Hot/Cold.** If you've got a "hot" condition, you're liable to have a flushed, red face, fever, irritability, thirst for cold liquids, and a dark red tongue. Cold reveals itself as the following symptoms or conditions: a pale complexion, quiet, feels cold, lack of thirst or thirst for only hot liquids, localized pain, and diarrhea.

➤ **Excessive/Deficient.** An excessive condition means you've got too much of a good thing. You might observe louder voice, pain that is worse from pressure, heavy breathing, thick coating on the tongue, strong pulse. Deficient implies not enough. The patient is quiet, withdrawn, voice is soft, breathing is light, pain is better from pressure, little or no coating on the tongue, weak pulse.

As discussed at the beginning of the chapter, all of these symptoms could fit into Yin or Yang. It's a way to begin making sense out of things, and this symbol always seems to be relevant as it shows the ever-changing dynamics of us all living together in our world, as well as what happens within each one of our human bodies.

Imagine trying to stay healthy and make some sense out of a topsy-turvy world. Sound like yesterday? Now you can see how it was done thousands of years ago by observing the changes and correspondences in nature and humans. That is why most of the names have a reference to natural occurrences like wind and heat. You've covered a pretty good background of medical philosophy, and are now ready to dive in to the conditions that will most likely bring you to your acu-pro in the first place.

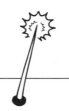

Acu-Moment

Your oriental practitioner will ideally tell you where the problem is, how you are doing, and suggest what to do about it. For example, here is how he or she would diagnose the condition called "Wind-Cold-Damp Headache."

Wind—Pain comes on quickly and can move around

Cold—Worse in cold, better with heat

Damp—Feels heavy, may also be digestive weakness

Headache—Good news! It's all in your head!

The Least You Need to Know

➤ An Oriental Medical diagnosis tells you what's going on and how your body is reacting.

➤ Keep your qi and blood brothers healthy and happy to avoid illness.

➤ Keep the weather conditions on the outside and not the inside.

➤ Stuck emotions can eventually lead to sickness.

Part 2

Stop the Pain Drain

Being in pain can feel like the life is being sucked out of you. Pain changes your world, whether it's an acute back sprain or debilitating chronic pain. To see how widespread pain is for you and your neighbors, just watch the commercials on television. According to Credit Suisse First Boston Corporation, $7.7 billion is spent worldwide for pain relief, and the number is growing by 7 percent a year. Americans spend over $3 billion dollars a year in over-the-counter pain medications, and $750 million for prescription pain sales. It was also estimated that there are 40 million doctor visits made each year because patients complained of pain.

The American Pain Society states that 45 percent of Americans seek medical help for persistent pain sometime in their lives. They go on to note that 68 percent of people with moderate to severe pain have used complementary/ alternative medical therapies for relief.

This part of the book deals with real solutions for pain from head to foot. We'll start at the top and work our way down through headaches, back pain, and foot pain. I believe the outlook for oriental medical therapies is promising in regard to stopping the pain drain on you and your family. So keep on reading … hope is just a few chapters away!

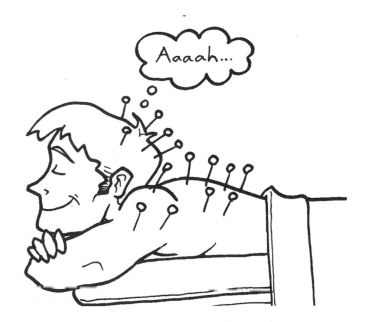

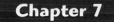

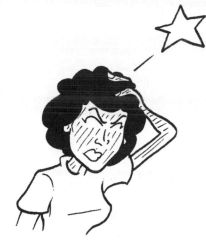

Chapter 7

Pain from the Neck Up

In This Chapter

➤ Relief from the horrors of headaches

➤ Solutions for post–op tooth pain

➤ A pain in the neck no longer

➤ Stop the pain and fatigue of fibromyalgia

Some days, when the pain of a headache gets bad, do you feel like unscrewing your head and asking for a refund? Hopefully you won't need to do that after reading this chapter on pain from the neck up. We'll be discussing some of the most common pains that occur above the neck, and then look at the ways that oriental medicine identifies what's going on and treats it. Headaches, dental and neck pain, and fibromyalgia are open for your examination. So hold onto your hat (and your head) while you learn valuable tips for taking the dread out of your head.

Headaches: Riot on the Rooftop!

If you suffer from headaches, you're not alone. According to the American Council for Headache Education, an estimated 50 million Americans experience some form of severe headache. About 26 million Americans have migraine headaches, either with an *aura* (classic migraine) or without (common migraine).

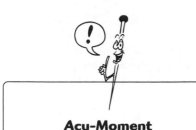

Migraines are the most common cause of recurring headaches, but other conditions can cause your head to ache as well, including high blood pressure, glaucoma, or sinusitis. Less likely causes are cerebral tumors and meningitis. Your acu-pro can work with your conventional physician to ensure everyone fully understands—from both a western and eastern perspective—what's causing your head to throb before you begin treatment.

Serious Sinus Relief

With your sinuses plugged and your head and face throbbing, this Cinderella is in no shape for the ball! Your sinus cavities are swollen and can't drain fluids properly … you've just been diagnosed with sinusitis.

Your acu-pro will examine you to find out what to do about your symptoms and help you stop the recurring sinus problems. In traditional oriental medicine, excess dampness is often the underlying cause of sinus problems. The feelings of heaviness, unclear thinking, a full feeling in the chest or stomach, and lack of appetite all point to dampness. Your acupuncturist will use acupoints that open up the sinus cavities and help them drain. He or she will also help you improve your digestion with food choices, herbs to keep the sinuses clear, and dry up the dampness.

> **Acu-Moment**
>
> An **aura** is a group of nerve symptoms experienced by approximately 5 percent of migraine sufferers. About 20–60 minutes before the headache, you may start to see things like flashing lights or zigzag lines, or experience partial loss of vision. Typically, an aura lasts between 10 and 25 minutes.

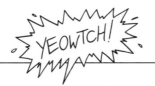

> **Harm Alarm**
>
> Watch out for the rebound! One of the most common causes of chronic daily headaches is an analgesic rebound headache. Taking analgesics (painkillers) on a daily basis or consuming excessive amounts of caffeine (coffee and soda are common culprits) are clues. The headaches occur when the medication wears off, prompting you to take more. Write down the times when you take medication and look at the cycle; you may be causing your own headaches.

Pressure Points to Take the Ache Out

Most of the points used here will also be used by your acu-pro. Here's how you can continue the treatment by continuing these acupressure techniques at home.

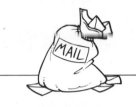

Mailbag

Simone worked as an office manager in a small company. She knew everyone and was on a first name basis with all the customers. She could coordinate the activities of multiple executives because they all knew each other's needs so well. When her chronic headaches kept her out of work, or she had to lie down in a darkened office for several hours, the office was a wreck. She came in with a diagnosis of migraine headaches for which she had taken numerous prescriptions and over-the-counter medications for years without satisfaction. We began a series of acupuncture sessions twice a week for three weeks to see if the results gave us both confidence to continue. By the second week she noticed a significant reduction in both the frequency and intensity of her headaches. Following the third week she had almost a whole week without pain and was learning to do home acupressure. She continues to work at a job where she is wanted and appreciated and has gone on to live a happier, more fulfilled life.

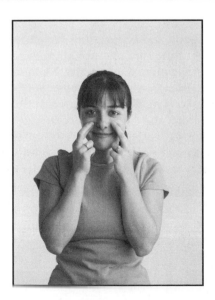

Relieving sinus headaches.

For sinus headaches, use your index and middle fingers to press firmly on LI-20 (Welcome Fragrance) located beside your nostrils. Close your eyes and concentrate while you press for two to three minutes, breathing deeply through your nose.

Headache relief.

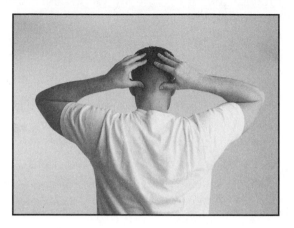

For headaches in the back of the head and neck, use your thumbs to press firmly into GB-20 (Pool of Wind). Tilt your head up as you feel for the hollow spots on the base of your skull, located on either side of the spine. Use your fingers for support and stability while you gently press for two minutes. Breathe deeply.

Dental Pain: Page the Tooth Fairy

Dental pain can be a troubling ordeal. If your teeth are in pain, you can scarcely take a comfortable breath. Your dentist should be consulted to help you discover the source of your pain.

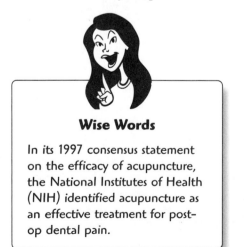

Wise Words

In its 1997 consensus statement on the efficacy of acupuncture, the National Institutes of Health (NIH) identified acupuncture as an effective treatment for post-op dental pain.

Acupuncture and acupressure have been shown to be effective in the treatment of alleviating toothaches and postoperative dental pain. I frequently treat patients after they've had oral surgery or teeth pulled (even all four wisdom teeth!). With the help of acupuncture, the pain and swelling go down much more quickly. Patients are able to return to work or regular household life much faster and with greater comfort.

Your acupuncturist may use electricity attached to the needles to increase the pain relief to your teeth. Don't be surprised if acu-points are used in your ears or feet to help bring down your pain.

Gentle Dental Acu-Points

The following acu-points have as their area of influence the teeth, jaw, and gum regions. These points can be coordinated with your acu-pro and dentist to ensure the most effective self-care treatments.

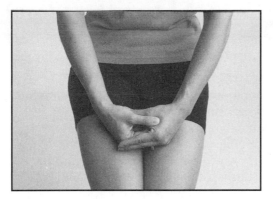

Relieving dental pain.

LI-4 (Adjoining Valleys) is located in the muscle between your thumb and index finger. Find the sore spot in the muscle next to the web of your hand on the same side as your sore tooth. Wrap your fingers around your hand while pressing firmly with your thumb. This point will probably be very sore, so be gentle. You can use this point while in the waiting room or dental chair. It will help relieve the pain and relax your body.

Relieving dental pain.

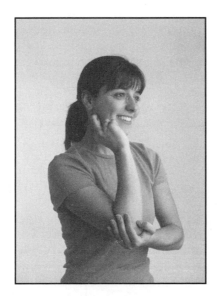

Find the corner of your jawbone and feel for sore acu-points as you go toward your mouth. Hold your thumbs under your jaw for support and, using your index and middle fingers, gently press for one to two minutes the points you found, probably ST-6 (Jaw Vehicle) or ST-7 (Lower Hinge). Close your eyes and take long, deep breaths.

Neck Pain: Release the Weight of the World

Your head weighs about 10–15 pounds. Your neck's job is to hold your head upright, all day, every day, which makes it a prime area for your body to hold stress, resulting in knotted cords of iron where your soft and subtle neck muscles used to be.

Today many people sit at desks or computers that are not set up ergonomically to work with your body. Unnecessary muscular tension results from long hours and emotional stress. Your neck is frequently a spot that is injured during sports or automobile accidents (see Chapter 10, "Injuries—Taking the Ouch out of the Oops!"). Chronic neck pain results when an injury is neglected, incompletely healed, or daily stress is allowed to build up over time.

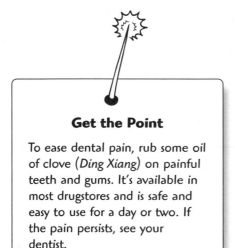

Get the Point

To ease dental pain, rub some oil of clove (*Ding Xiang*) on painful teeth and gums. It's available in most drugstores and is safe and easy to use for a day or two. If the pain persists, see your dentist.

Your acu-pro will look for pain patterns that correspond to oriental diagnostic patterns such as dampness (heavy, dull ache, worse on rainy days), stuck blood (fixed, stabbing pain), or wind (pain moves around from side to side). Depending on the pattern, look for him or her to use acupuncture, moxibustion, or Tui-Na, and to teach you self-care techniques such Qi Gong, acupressure, and nutritional support. Neck pain from many different causes can be successfully treated with Oriental Medicine.

Stop the Neck Wreck

Since you will not be seeing your acu-pro everyday, here are some points to press whenever the spirit or the stress moves you. Self-care is an important component in staying healthy and the following guidelines are designed to do throughout your day when a quick health break and deep breathing will do you good.

Let your hands rest on either side of your jaw, so that the middle finger touches GB-20 (Pool of Wind) at the base of your skull. Tilt your head slightly up and press deeply and firmly into the hollow places with your middle finger. Tilt your head downward and begin to rub down either side of your spine in small firm circles. Make sure to take long, deep breaths and to stop longer at extra-sore points. Repeat several times to release chronic stiffness.

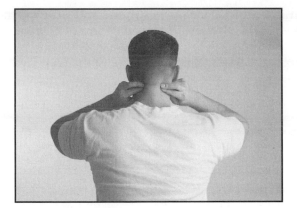

Relieving neck pain and stiffness.

Fibromyalgia: Tired of Being Sick and Tired

Myalgia (muscle pain) characterizes this often-devastating chronic rheumatic pain disorder of unknown cause. The pain is usually described as "achy," but a few patients tell me they can also experience burning, throbbing, stabbing, or shooting pain. To make this dish sound even more appetizing, fibromyalgia is often accompanied by side orders of chronic headaches, strange skin sensations, temporomandibular joint pain (TMJ), insomnia, irritable bowel syndrome (IBS), anxiety, palpitations, fatigue, poor memory, painful menstruation, and depression.

Diagnosing fibromyalgia is difficult because we don't know what causes this condition. Patients are often frustrated because they have met many physicians who say, "It's all in your head." There have been links to the onset of symptoms and exposure to Epstein-Barr virus (EBV) that causes mononucleosis. Since pain and fatigue are key symptoms, others have thought it may be connected to chronic fatigue syndrome (CFS).

Fibromyalgia occurs mostly in women, many of whom have experienced insomnia, anxiety, stress, or depression along with the muscle aches. The symptoms are often severe enough to greatly interrupt their normal life and, in many cases, patients are unable to stay at work or continue normal household activities like cooking, childcare, or shopping.

Treating fibromyalgia successfully requires a consistent and sustained approach by both the patient and acu-pro. I have been pleased to have helped many patients regain their lives, but it took both of us working together with spouses, friends, and

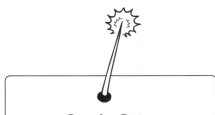

Get the Point

Sigh and the world sighs with you! Sighing out loud on an exhalation helps to further release tight muscles as you perform acupressure. The sigh makes sure you are taking in enough air, which helps to oxygenate sore muscles and help release emotional stress and worry that may contribute to your aches and pains. All together now, say "Aaaaah!"

conventional physicians, creating a true balance of healthcare and self-care. In oriental medical theory, most of the patients I've seen have some form of cold-damp-wind pain. This name implies that the pain gets worse with cold, better with heat; is characterized by poor digestion and achy, heavy, tired muscles; and the pain changes location between the tender points.

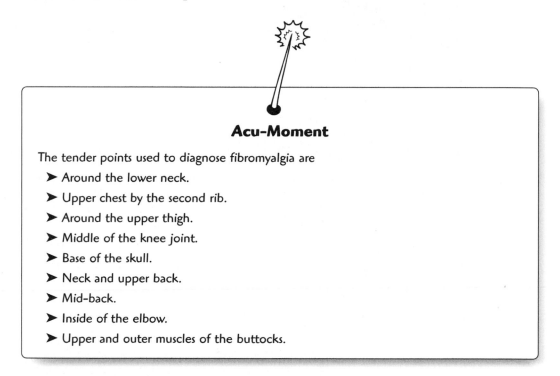

Acu-Moment

The tender points used to diagnose fibromyalgia are

➤ Around the lower neck.

➤ Upper chest by the second rib.

➤ Around the upper thigh.

➤ Middle of the knee joint.

➤ Base of the skull.

➤ Neck and upper back.

➤ Mid-back.

➤ Inside of the elbow.

➤ Upper and outer muscles of the buttocks.

Acupuncture, massage, and Chinese herbal medicine are recommended as effective treatments by the Fibromyalgia Network (see Appendix D, "State and National Organizations"). The Network is an organization that provides information to patients with this potentially debilitating condition. Moxi-bustion or infrared heat treatments are also useful in driving out the cold. Nutritional supplements such as antioxidants (coenzyme Q10, vitamins E and C) are helpful in managing this condition, as are dietary changes to eliminate dampness and build immunity.

Render Tender Points Painless

Any of the tender points can be pressed with slow, gradual pressure while breathing deeply for one to two minutes.

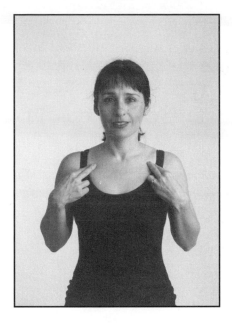

Relieving tender points.

Feel around for a sore spot at the end of your clavicle or collarbone, LU-1 (Central Residence). With your fingers in a loose fist resting against your chest, use reinforced fingers, breath deeply, and hold these points for two to three minutes. Mild pressure may be applied as you exhale; release as you inhale. This will invigorate your neck muscles and stimulate circulation in your lungs.

Now that you've got the top part of your body in better shape let's move on to the rest. I have always felt it's better to have options in treating conditions such as headaches, dental, and neck pain. Fibromyalgia has also responded so favorably to treatment that I had to include it in the text. Go ahead to the next chapter to begin experiencing the relief for some of the most common shoulder and joint pains.

The Least You Need to Know

➤ Acupuncture gives serious sinus relief.

➤ The National Institutes of Health (NIH) suggests acupuncture shows evidence for helping post-op dental pain.

➤ Say "no way" to neck pain through acupressure.

➤ Oriental Medicine holds help for fibromyalgia sufferers.

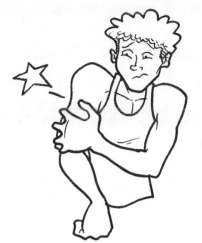

Chapter 8

Keeping Pain at Arm's Length

In This Chapter

➤ Acu-therapy to bounce back from bursitis

➤ Stop courting the pain of tennis elbow

➤ Learn the stretches and catches to combat carpal tunnel

➤ Discover time-tested techniques to ease arthritic pain and suffering

---

Some of the most prolific and common pains occur along the joints that lie from the shoulder to the fingers. These joints are pretty "handy" because we rely on them constantly throughout the day to help us dress, drive our cars, do our laundry, and hold our babies.

When you experience pain in any of the joints of your arms, it makes it hard to do most anything. Most activities become a struggle. With shoulder bursitis, you can hardly comb your own hair. Tennis elbow makes it a challenge to pick up a pot full of water off your stove. Carpal tunnel limits your productivity at work, and arthritis in your hands can seem like an impregnable barrier to any task.

The good news is that Oriental Medicine has been aiding the healing of joint pain for centuries. This chapter will focus on the treatments and self-care options to help you keep pain at arm's length—and more. Keep turning these pages to discover the acu-advantage for yourself.

Bursitis: The Cursa the Bursa

Bursitis is an inflammation of the bursae, which are the saclike capsules that surround joints such as the elbow, knee, or hip. The sacs are filled with thick liquid used to literally lubricate the joint and cut down on friction. When the tissue around the sacs becomes inflamed, your joints are painful to move and you start looking like the Tin Man from *The Wizard of Oz*—your joints feel stiff and each of your movements is accompanied by pain. Luckily, by using acu-points to lube up your bursa, you won't feel the worsa.

Shoulder Bursitis: Play Ball (Again!)

Bursitis of the shoulder is by far the most common. Trauma from a sports injury or chronic overuse is usually at the root of it all. If your shoulder does not heal on its own, acu-pros have a good track record at getting you back in the game.

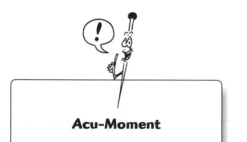

Acu-Moment

Bursitis, the inflammation of the saclike capsules that surround joints, has been around for a long time, and many of the common names reflect the occupations that suffered most from it. Examples include miner's elbow, housemaid's knee, and tailor's, or weaver's bottom.

In traditional Oriental Medicine, the symptoms of bursitis translate to the pattern of stuck blood. The pain is often sharp and fixed in one spot and temporarily feels worse when you press on that spot. Common local points include LI-15 (Shoulder Bone), TH-14 (Shoulder Seam), and Jianneiling (Shoulder's Inner Tomb), an extra point off the main channel system. (They really have the shoulder theme going strong here!) Your acupuncturist may use needle, electromagnetic, or electroauricular acupuncture to get the blood moving again and decrease inflammation in the joint. If you are typically cold by nature or your shoulder feels better with warmth, your acu-pro may choose to use moxibustion (see Chapter 5, "Acupuncture—Tools of the Trade"). Cupping jars or magnets (also see Chapter 5) may also be appropriate to free up your shoulder. Most of these are non-needle techniques, but all can help clear up pain in your shoulder.

Acupressure self-care uses firm but steady pressure on these acu-points to press the inflammation out of the tissues and bring new blood to that tired old sac. I'll show you some of the most frequently used points, but I encourage you to feel for tender points around the joint. Try to move your shoulder and press where you feel it holds you back. Use a firm and steady pressing method with either thumb or reinforced index finger on all points. Press while exhaling for 10–15 breaths.

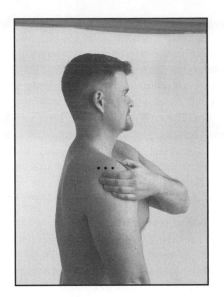

With thumb or reinforced index finger, press deeply into the joint with as much pressure as you can manage. Breathe deeply for 10–15 breaths as you slowly move the shoulder.

Move It or Lose It

A common reaction to painful shoulder bursitis is to hold it still and hope that it gets better on its own. It may, but odds are you are only making things worse by allowing the muscles to weaken and inflammation to set up shop. Reestablishing your normal range of motion and strength is vital. You ought to be able to put on a jacket, reach the top shelf for a glass, or tuck in your shirt without severe pain. Start with mild arm swings that slowly and gently move your shoulder joint. As your pain reduces, increase the height of the arm swing until you can comfortably lift it above your shoulder.

Tennis Elbow: The Gripes of the Grip

You certainly don't have to be playing tennis to experience the nagging and often disabling pain on the outside of your elbow that we commonly call tennis elbow. Tennis elbow, or lateral humeral epicondylitis, usually results from overuse of this joint, either on the tennis court or elsewhere. When patients talk about what was going on prior to the pain, typically there's a history of mini-aches or twinges around the bone that's on the outside of the elbow.

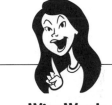

Wise Words

White Crane Qi Gong imitates the soft and balanced movements of the white crane's wings. These practices can benefit the shoulder and upper back by increasing your motion without the notion of pain. Soft, gentle movements combined with deep breathing create a relaxed way to efficiently move and gradually strengthen your shoulder. When you become truly proficient, who knows—maybe you'll be able to fly to your next appointment!

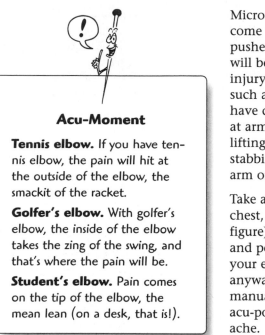

Acu-Moment

Tennis elbow. If you have tennis elbow, the pain will hit at the outside of the elbow, the smackit of the racket.

Golfer's elbow. With golfer's elbow, the inside of the elbow takes the zing of the swing, and that's where the pain will be.

Student's elbow. Pain comes on the tip of the elbow, the mean lean (on a desk, that is!).

Microtears in the muscle over time mean you'll feel it come on slowly, unless a single occasion of overuse pushes you over the edge into severe pain. The pain will be worse during and after use. Depending on the injury, you may experience pain only with activities such as tennis. In a more advanced condition, you'll have difficulty with any task where you hold objects at arm's length, such as pouring from a juice carton or lifting a pot off the stove. The pain is often sharp and stabbing in nature and can send zings into your forearm or hand.

Take a moment to place your bent arm around your chest, as if you were in an arm sling (see the following figure). Feel the bony bump on the side of your elbow and poke around in front of the bone (going toward your elbow crease) for a sore spot. This may feel achy anyway, but if you have been overdoing it with a manual screwdriver or playing tennis too often, this acu-point will probably be a little worse than a minor ache.

Tennis elbow is a commonly treated condition in my clinic. Successful outcome and patient satisfaction are usually high. Oriental diagnosis of tennis elbow is stuck Qi or blood (pain ranging from dull and achy to sharp and stabbing). Treatment involves the use of needle acupuncture, electroacupuncture, and non-needle options such as electromagnetic or biomagnetic acupuncture.

Moxibustion is used if the pain is chronic, or if the patient feels an increase in discomfort with cold or damp weather. You can expect the practitioner to apply pressure to acu-points around the elbow as well as along the Qi channel (bicep, forearm, and hand) to increase circulation and decrease pain. Resting or cutting back on activities that worsen pain is the common-sense prescription, but because these actions often involve daily activities, resting the joint is not always possible. However, your acu-pro will work to speed up the healing of the elbow using acupressure techniques.

Acupressure: The Match Points

Acupressure is an effective and timesaving technique for healing tennis elbow. The acu-points are located along the channels that affect the outside of the elbow. As you'll see by their names, these acu-points are famous for treating elbows just like yours.

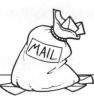

Mailbag

Len came to the office in desperation. He wanted to keep playing in his tennis league and be able to hold the phone or type at work. I immediately suggested he get a headset for his office and asked him to cut back on all unnecessary tennis. You'd have thought it was a death sentence. He reluctantly agreed to the tennis part to avoid further aggravation of his condition. He was taking prescription medication from his physician, but that had not helped. We began treatment consisting of electromagnetic acupuncture, home acupressure and biomagnetic treatments with ice and a topical homeopathic ointment named Rhuta Graveolus. His pain and stiffness began to consistently lessen. He tried to go back to his original schedule too soon and re-injured his elbow. The setback is not uncommon, but added another two weeks of treatment time to correct. He now is able to do what he wants and cuts back a little to do his home treatments when his discomfort increases.

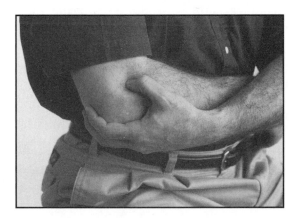

These points will be tender, making them easier to find. Apply a combination of deep penetrating thumb pressure for one to three minutes, followed by slow counterclockwise rubbing of the acu-points.

Use these ocu-points to relieve tennis elbow:

➤ LI-11 (Crooked Pool)—Located midway between the tip of the bone on the outside of the elbow and the end of the crease in the elbow that's closest to the bone

➤ LI-12 (Elbow Seam)—Located one finger width above LI-11

➤ LI-10 (Arm's Three Measures)—Located two-finger width below LI-11 on the forearm

➤ Ashi Point—Located anyplace around the outside of the elbow that's sore

Another technique to use on tennis elbow is the cross fiber Tui-Na pushing.

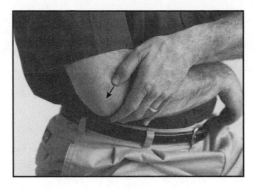

Find the sore spot in the elbow and gently, but firmly apply steady pressure as you push toward the bone on the outside of the elbow. Repeat three to four strokes at a time once or twice a day. This will contribute to decreasing inflammation and pain.

Carpal Tunnel Syndrome: The Mouse That Made You Roar

Carpal tunnel syndrome is named after the tube or tunnel that passes through the carpal bones (hence the name "carpal") in the heel of the hand. The prime pain spot is located in the area where the hand meets the wrist. If the size of the tunnel is reduced, pressure is put on the median nerve, producing the characteristic numbness and pain of carpal tunnel syndrome.

Let's take a look. Turn your palm toward you, tilt your palm toward your face, make a fist, and squeeze. Do you see the tendons that pop up and run like side-by-side railroad tracks from your wrist to your hand? The median nerve is underneath these tendons. When it's pinched, you hurt.

Carpal tunnel syndrome has become famous as a work-related, repetitive strain injury (see Chapter 10, "Injuries—Taking the Ouch out of the Oops!"), but more than half of all patients cannot trace their condition to a particular activity.

Trouble in the Tunnel

Symptoms of carpal tunnel syndrome often crop up after you start a new job or a new hobby that forces you to use your wrist and fingers in a repetitive motion. Women are particularly susceptible to developing the condition, especially if they're pregnant or between the ages of 40 and 70. The pain can affect one or both arms and can involve pain in the forearm, wrist, and/or palm. Some patients with carpal tunnel feel a sharp pain when they make the repetitive movement, others experience a constant numbness or tingling in the thumb, index, middle, and half of the ring finger.

The symptoms often worsen at night, and can get so bad that the patient has to wake up in order to shake his or her hands to relieve the numbness. If you're affected by carpal tunnel syndrome, you may also have difficulty with fine motor skills, such as writing or crocheting, and you may find yourself dropping things from the affected hand.

The Terminator in the Tunnel: Acupuncture on the Scene

In traditional Oriental Medical terms, the symptoms of carpal tunnel syndrome reflect cold (a victim often feels more pain with cold), dampness (forearm and hand may feel heavy and achy), and wind (characterizes the tingling or shooting nerve pain) that block the otherwise smooth flow of blood and Qi in our arms.

Acupuncture treatments include stimulation of acu-points near the wrist by an in-and-out technique with the needle. You may feel a mild electrical sensation, which is desired because it will help release the tendons and decrease pain and numbness. Acupuncture needles, electroacupuncture, electromagnetic acupuncture, moxibustion, magnet therapy, and even laser acupuncture are successfully used in treating carpal tunnel syndrome.

In addition to receiving treatment from your acu-pro, you should avoid activities that might aggravate your wrists, such as prolonged writing with a pen, working at a computer, performing assembly line work, or even working as a trapeze artist! If you sleep with your wrists curled up under your chin or pillow, your acu-pro may suggest a nighttime splint to keep you from further damaging your wrists while you sleep.

I'll Be Back: Acupressure Stretch and Press

Acupressure is a great self-care treatment that speeds up recovery time and can be used to break up the tension in your wrists at work. The following exercises can really help relieve your suffering.

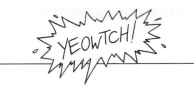

Harm Alarm

Don't assume it's carpal tunnel syndrome. Other conditions, such as diabetes, alcoholism, wrist fractures, and arthritis of the sixth vertebra in the neck, have similar symptoms. Check with your health professional to rule out these or other conditions.

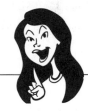

Wise Words

Margaret Naeser, Ph.D., licensed acupuncturist and associate research professor of neurology at the Boston University School of Medicine, has been using low-energy lasers (5–20 megawatts compared to a typical surgical laser of 300 watts) to treat post-surgical pain from carpal tunnel syndrome. A red beam is all you see on your wrist or hand. You don't feel a thing while you end the zing!

*Relieving carpal tunnel
syndrome.*

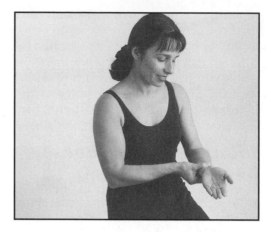

Apply firm and steady pressure for one to three minutes to the acu-points that follow the median nerve and flexor tendons into the hand. Acu-points include P-6 (Inner Gate), located between the two tendons, two-finger width from the wrist; P-7 (Big Tomb), located midpoint of the crease that runs across the wrist; and P-8 (Labor's Palace), located in the middle of the palm between the second and third bones of the hand (between the index and middle fingers).

*Relieving carpal tunnel
syndrome.*

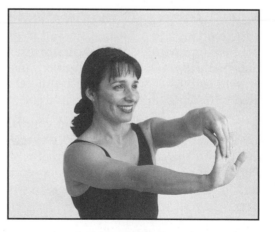

While keeping your arm out straight and your hand in good alignment with your arm, pull straight back to achieve a steady, even, gentle stretch of the carpal tunnel region. Pull back for 2–3 seconds while exhaling, and repeat this 6–10 times in one session. Remember to limit the pulling to just 2–3 seconds. Repeat the whole set once or twice daily.

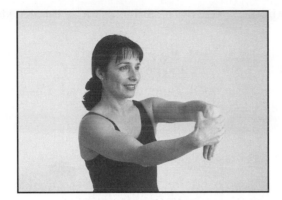

This exercise is exactly like the one in the preceding figure except you are stretching the top of the wrist that is often sore and contracted from the extra load of compensating for weakened inner wrist muscles. Repeat the same procedures.

Arthritis: Speakin' of the Creakin'

Arthritis is the common name given to a host of conditions that affect the joints. More than 50 million Americans suffer from some form of arthritis. We're born with lots of different joints in our body that allow us to move about easily, but when arthritis hits, the characteristic stiffness and pain can simply stop you in your tracks.

Causes of the Creakin'

There are a number of different types of arthritis, including

➤ **Osteoarthritis.** Average age at onset: over 40. Characteristics: gradual stiffness and pain, enlargement of the joint.

➤ **Rheumatoid arthritis.** Average age at onset: 25–50. Characteristics: autoimmune condition (immune system cells kill body cells), inflammation of the joint and neighboring tendons, muscles, and nerves.

➤ **Spondyloarthropathies.** Average age at onset: 20–40. Characterisitics: spinal inflammation and pain, often causing postural changes.

➤ **Gout.** Average age at onset: 40–43. Characteristics: sudden severe pain and swelling of a large joint, usually the big toe.

➤ **Lupus.** Average age at onset: 18–50. Characteristics: fever, weakness, facial and joint pain.

➤ **Juvenile rheumatoid arthritis.** Average age at onset: under 18. Characteristics: autoimmune

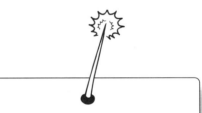

Get the Point

Get right into an "herbal soup" to soothe your aching joints. Place 9–12 grams of cinnamon (Gui Zhi), fresh ginger (Sheng Jiang), dried peach kernel (Tao Ren), and milk vetch root (Huang Qi) in a pot. Cover with water, bring to a boil, simmer 10 minutes, and strain off the water. After it has cooled down, place your stiff hands in the container and massage the warm herbal liquid into your joints. You can reboil and use the herbs and water several times.

condition, stiffness (often in the knees, wrists, or hands). May involve kidneys, heart, lungs, and nervous system.

➤ **Infectious arthritis.** Average age at onset: any. Characteristics: body aches, chills, fever, low blood pressure, swelling and pain that spread to other joints.

➤ **Kawasaki syndrome.** Average age at onset: 6 months to 11 years. Characteristics: fever, joint pain, rash on palms and soles, and heart problems.

Oriental Aids for Arthritis

Arthritis in its many forms is a common condition to be treated by Oriental Medicine. Your acu-pro will determine which environmental factor affects you: wind (moving pain), dampness (localized heavy ache), cold (worse from exposure to cold temperatures), or heat (skin is swollen, inflamed, and hot to the touch). He or she will treat the specific areas of your complaint and help improve your general health to keep you feeling good.

Acupuncture is widely used for arthritis and has served my patients well over the years. There are currently studies being conducted on several sites of arthritis being treated by acupuncture, such as knee osteoarthritis. I use a diverse mix of acupuncture techniques including the traditional needle system and electromagnetic acupuncture. All have their place in a series of treatments when determining which one or combination will give the most relief. Moxibustion is used to warm acu-points and channels, relieving the cold aches, while acupuncture in all its forms moves stuck blood and Qi to increase flexibility and decrease pain.

Acupressure and Tui-Na massage will use firm pressure over tender arthritic nodules and sore ashi points along the muscles and joints. Nodules are the hard, tender lumps you find in muscles and acu-points.

Qi Gong exercises are often taught to patients. The slow, gradual movements and deep breathing help keep joints moving and increase circulation. Food therapy and Chinese herbal medicine are effectively used to nourish your body, treat any underlying problems, and keep you feeling good. Arthritis is one of the conditions that Oriental Medicine has been treating for centuries. See your acu-pro to discover what kind of help is waiting for you.

Feeling better? Little by little, we'll cover many of the health concerns that you have, and you can even pick up some tips for your friends. So far you've gotten some solid solutions to such nagging complaints as tennis elbow, bursitis, carpal tunnel, and arthritis. You've got stretches, acu-points, and herbs to chew on. What's next? Your lower torso awaits to get on the healing path.

> ### The Least You Need to Know
>
> ➤ Acupuncture relieves swollen, painful bursitis.
>
> ➤ Firm acupressure on LI-12, LI-11, or LI-10 can reduce tennis elbow pain.
>
> ➤ Electro- or laser acupuncture short-circuits carpal tunnel pain and numbness.
>
> ➤ Make an "herbal soup" to wash away your arthritic pain and stiffness.

Chapter 9

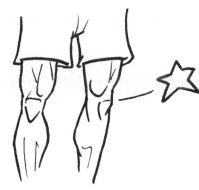

Pain Below the Belt

In This Chapter

➤ Acu-points that give relieve from back pain

➤ A low-back stretch to keep you limber and loose

➤ Stop the burning pain of sciatica

➤ End the pain of popping knees with Oriental Medicine

➤ Take a confident step by using acu-pros for foot pain

"Hitting below the belt" is an old sports expression for an unfair move. There's nothing fair about the conditions discussed in this chapter, because they can force you to take an unwanted timeout. Back pain can certainly sideline you, while sciatica should be a foul because it's literally a pain in the butt. Many of us are caught "traveling" around with sore and painful knees, while plantar fasciitis is roughing the kicker, runner, or walker with unneeded foot pain.

Luckily, you can get your acu-pro to play on your team and bring some time-tested game plans that have helped players like you stay in the thick of things. Turn the page and let's play ball!

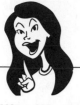

Oh, My Aching Back

If you've ever had back pain, then none of these statistics will probably surprise you. The Mayo Foundation estimates that four out of five adults will experience back pain in their lives. Back pain is the leading cause of disability for people between the ages of 19 and 45. When your back hurts, there is hardly any position or movement that is comfortable.

A few causes of back pain include the following:

Acute

➤ Overuse

➤ Improper lifting

➤ Kidney infection

Chronic

➤ Arthritis

➤ Overcurvature of the spine

➤ Overweight

➤ Sleeping on your stomach

➤ Sleeping on an old mattress

➤ Worn-out shoes

➤ Poor posture

➤ Constipation

➤ Kidney, bladder, or prostate problems

➤ Bone diseases and herniated disks

➤ Weak abdominal and back muscles

The good news is that acupuncture has proven to be an effective reliever of back pain, and acupressure techniques are some of the best ways to care for your own back. Weekend warriors that wake up the morning after with a stiff back will love the relief and shortened recovery time these techniques provide.

If you have a kidney infection—a serious condition—you will feel pain on only one side in the small of your back, feel generally sick, and have a fever. Consult your health professional immediately to clarify the origin of your pain if you are unclear.

Treating chronic pain usually involves modifying some old habits. Take a look at your posture. Try sitting with both feet flat on the floor in an upright, relaxed position. Examine the soles of your shoes. Are they worn on one side, showing how you are off balance when you walk? Start a new awareness and go out and buy a new pair of shoes.

In traditional Oriental Medical terms, acute low-back pain is the result of stuck Qi and blood (sharp pain in one place). Chronic low-back pain may be an excess of dampness (heavy, achy) or wind (pain moves around). If the pain has been there awhile, there is almost always a lack of circulation of Qi and blood, along with a weakening of the yin and yang energies of the surrounding organs. Difficulties with your bowels and urinary tract system will point your acu-pro in the best direction possible to help your back and entire body feel good.

Acu-points for treating back pain are located along the bladder channel. This particular channel runs from your head to your toes. A kink in this channel can definitely cramp your style. The acu-points used to heal the low back include BL-23 (Kidney's Hollow), BL-47 (The Will's Dwelling), CV-6 (Sea of Qi), and BL-54 (Commission the Middle). BL-23 and BL-47 are located in the small of the back. They are two and four fingers away from the center of the spine level, with the second and third lumbar vertebrae. CV-6 is two-finger width directly below your belly button, and BL-54 is found in the center of the crease behind your knee.

Your acupuncturist may choose a variety of techniques to treat your low-back pain, depending on the Oriental Medical diagnosis. Don't be surprised if your practitioner uses heat in the form of moxa or infrared heat therapy, especially if you hurt the most when you are cold. Relax and imagine you're on the beach in the sun. Traditional needle acupuncture, electroacupuncture, or electromagnetic acupuncture or cupping may be used on these points (see the techniques discussed in Chapter 5, "Acupuncture—Tools of the Trade").

Acupressure self-care for low-back pain is easy to learn, and the reward is feeling good the more you practice. Pay close attention to hand positions and point locations at first. Then let your fingers find the sore spots and enjoy the changes as your back relaxes.

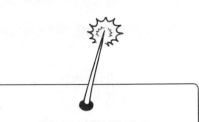

Get to the Point

Drink lots of water if you suffer from sudden low-back strain. It's often the result of overwork, resulting in a buildup of lactic acid in your muscles. One or two 8-ounce glasses of water may bring relief in just a few minutes. Bottoms up!

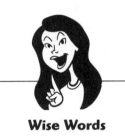

Wise Words

The **quadratus lumborum muscles** are the pillars of the low back. Muscle fibers connect the back of the hip to the 12th rib to stabilize and strengthen your low back and trunk.

You can stimulate BL-54 by placing your fingertips in the center of the creases behind your knees and either pressing deeply or rubbing while exhaling. This point stimulates lymphatic circulation that carries away inflammation from tired and sore muscles in your back. You can rub these points while at home, at dinner with friends, or at the movies. With the smile that'll be on your face, you might start a new craze!

I don't think I'm "stretching" the truth when I tell you that after your back muscles have been drained of their tension, a good stretch can keep you free of pain. I've found the main muscle in low-back pain is often a sturdy friend who is just worn out—the *quadratus lumborum*. Here's an exercise to relieve your back of its tension and pain.

Caring for low-back pain.

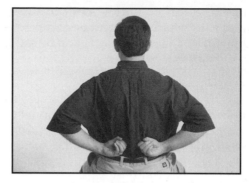

Lightly place loose fists on BL-23 or BL-47 with the thumb and index finger touching your back. Rub fists in a quick clockwise direction so they generate heat, breathe deeply, and continue for one minute.

Caring for low-back pain.

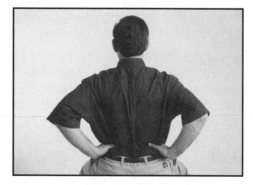

Using your thumbs, press BL-23 or BL-47 directly into the back or toward the spine. Search for tight, stringing muscles and press deeply while exhaling two or three breaths for each point.

Relieving the tension in the back.

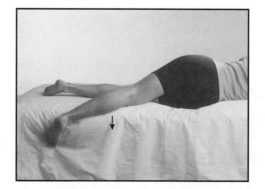

Lie on an elevated table or bed, letting the top leg hang behind the lower leg. Breathe deeply and relax, allowing the weight of the leg to passively stretch the leg, hip, and low back.

Ice and heat can be great tools in your pursuit of pain-free living, but you've got to use them wisely. The chilling facts about ice are simple: Ice slows inflammation, lessens swelling, and alleviates pain. Apply it to the injury within the first 36–48 hours of sudden back pain. I know you like the idea of heat, but that comes later. During the third day of pain, if swelling is still present but reduced, you can alternate applying ice and heat. Always end with ice.

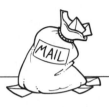

Mailbag

Ernie's primary care physician recommended that Ernie see me for treatment of severe low-back strain with sciatica extending down the right leg. Ernie works in a large retail company in the maintenance department where he typically is called upon to lift heavy objects and move them around all day. He takes pride in his work and did not like to just "sit around all day," but would rather like to do projects around his home. I saw Ernie during the winter months in New England when there is a certain need for a homeowner to shovel the white stuff and be steady on his feet. He always felt that he was going to slip on the ice and hurt himself even more. He had never tried anything like acupuncture, but wanted to feel better. We began treatment twice a week using needle acupuncture and infrared heat treatments. His pain was definitely worse in the cold. After the first week he felt enough improvement to be cautiously optimistic. We continued treatments and added acupressure techniques in the office and at home. Stretches were added the following week, and he began to experience consistent pain relief, improved sleep, and more confidence. His physician gave him an "okay" to return to work, and Ernie was able to stay at work and continue his home therapies to keep fit.

Finally, we come to heat—the favorite application on a cold winter night. If cold makes your pain worse, apply heat to help increase circulation. Make a healing sandwich by using a heating pad under your low back on BL-23/47, and a hot water bottle resting on CV-6 under your navel. Breathe deeply and visualize the heat loosening all your muscles and filling your body with energy.

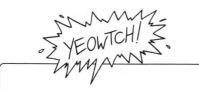

Harm Alarm

Avoid using acupressure on slipped, fractured, or disintegrating spinal discs. A trip to your medical, osteopathic, or chiropractic physician will identify the cause to be cured.

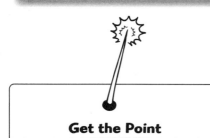

Get the Point

Tennis, anyone? You can use a tennis ball to stimulate acu-points on your back or hips. Locate the acu-point, such as GB-30 (Encircling Leap), place the ball at the point, then lay your body weight on top of the ball. Take several long, slow breaths as you allow the tennis ball to press into sore muscles for one to two minutes. Repeat one or two times a day, and you'll be sitting pretty!

Sciatica: The Nerve of It

Developing sciatica is unfair because you rarely get a break from its pain. The pain is present when you sit, stand, and even while you're lying down. Sciatica is the familiar term for pain that travels along the sciatic nerve, which starts in the middle of your butt, runs down the back of your leg, and sometimes extends to your foot. The farther down you feel the characteristic pain, burning, or numbness, the more pressure is being put on the root of the nerve in your butt.

What could cause this pressure? The most common cause is a herniated or slipped disk in your low back. Other causes include muscle spasms in the low back and hip (sacraliliac region and periformis) or intraspinal tumor. Checking with your primary care provider will ensure a proper diagnosis and the most effective treatment.

Oriental Medicine categorizes sciatica according to how you feel. The diagnostic category of wind is used for pain that moves around, while dampness characterizes the often stiff, heavy ache in the hip muscles. In traditional Chinese medicine terms, cold, stuck Qi and blood cause the sharp stabbing pain of sciatica.

During the past 15 years of my practice, I've felt that I've been most successful helping patients with sciatica get some relief. Patients will walk in leaning to one side to relieve the pressure on the nerve, and often walk out smiling and greatly improved.

Acupuncture stimulation is achieved by clicking on the *DaQi* or big Qi sensation switch. By that, I mean having a practitioner insert needles into acu-points and lifting or rotating them until you feel sensations such as electric current, warmth, or temporary achiness. These sensations let your acupuncturist know the channel switch is turned on and help is on the way. Typical techniques include needle acupuncture with electricity or moxa.

Elbow Your Pain Out of the Way

The sciatic nerve is located deep in the muscles of the buttocks, so the acupressure techniques used to reach the affected area need to penetrate through layers of muscles. If you used your fingers or thumbs, you'd be sore in a very short time. That is why acu-pros use their elbows or tools to stimulate the points and put an end to your pain.

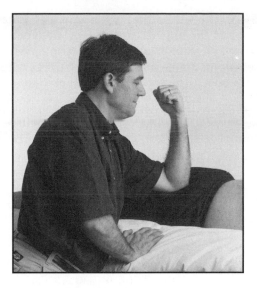

Elbowing the way to the sciatic nerve.

The main acu-point to use is GB-30 (Encircling Leap), which is located one-third the distance from your hipbone (Greater Trochanter) to your sacrum (the V-shaped bone below your back). Keep your body in proper alignment (body over hips, knees bent) as you place the tip of your elbow on the point of your willing subject. Lean your body into the point with firm and deep pressure for 30 seconds to 1 minute. Ask the person to breathe deeply. The point will be sore, so apply only as much pressure as the patient can comfortably stand.

Knee Pain: What's the Deal with Your Kneel?

Your knees are the joints that connect your body to your feet. They are central to distributing your body weight over your feet so that you can walk, run, ski, or jump. When you hear popping and creaking sounds from your knees, be calm, and thank your acu-pro for getting the healing started!

Get the Point

The knee is the largest and most complicated joint in your body. The knee is placed under tremendous stress while you walk, run, squat, or lift heavy objects. Many tendons and ligaments crisscross your knee like a Christmas-present bow to stabilize and give added strength to this out-of-sight, out-of-mind joint.

Our knees hold us up all our lives, and as time goes by, they become especially prone to injuries. Common diagnoses include arthritis, bursitis, and strains or tears of ligaments and tendons. Please select a qualified practitioner to help you discover the origin of your pain. Your acu-pro can help heal many of the strains and arthritic conditions. In my experience, ligament and tendon tears are only mildly improved with acupuncture and require conventional medical care such as surgery.

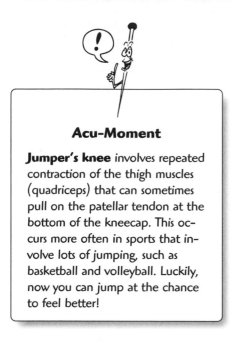

Acu-Moment

Jumper's knee involves repeated contraction of the thigh muscles (quadriceps) that can sometimes pull on the patellar tendon at the bottom of the kneecap. This occurs more often in sports that involve lots of jumping, such as basketball and volleyball. Luckily, now you can jump at the chance to feel better!

Most of the acu-points for the knee are located in the joint and the muscles that support the knee. Treatment is based on your experience with pain and will differ if the pain becomes worse with cold or is a constant, dull, heavy ache (damp) or is sharp (stuck Qi).

Techniques that increase circulation and decrease swelling and pain are used and may include using acupuncture needles, electricity, and electromagnetics. Chinese herbal medicine may be prescribed internally to deal with an overall damp and cold condition that aggravates the knee, or used in an external herbal wash (the warm liquid of boiled herbs rubbed on the surface of the knee with a washcloth).

Capping Off Knee Pain

Your kneecap, or patella, should move around easily when your weight is off your leg. There are two ligaments that hold it loosely in place right under the kneecap. If you sit in a chair with your feet flat on the floor, feel for the small indentations near the bottom of your kneecap on either side. These acu-points are located here at ST-35 and Xiyan (Eyes of Knee). This area can get swollen and sore, especially after sports activities involving jumping. Another name for this condition, patellar tendonitis, is *jumper's knee*.

Relieving patellar tendonitis, or jumper's knee.

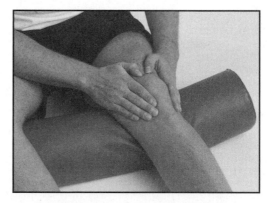

Sit on the floor to take the weight off your knee and feel your kneecap slide up and down and side to side. It should glide easily. If there is pain or it feels like you have speed bumps, have it checked out by your healthcare practitioner. Using your thumbs and fingers, feel around the outside edges of the kneecap for any sore spots. Press firmly for a minute or two while taking long, slow breaths. Rub and knead the area to increase blood and Qi flow.

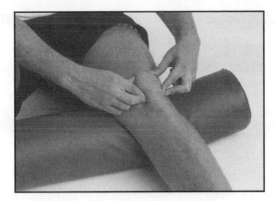

Relieving patellar tendonitis, or jumper's knee.

Place a pillow under your knees and support your back by leaning against a wall. Find the tender spots on the outside crease of your knee (lateral meniscus) and inside (medial meniscus). Use your index and middle fingers to press firmly for approximately one to two minutes per spot. Breathe deeply while rubbing vigorously with your palm afterward.

Plantar Fasciitis: A Step in the Right Direction

Feeling pain in your foot with every step you take? Now what? Plantar fasciitis is inflammation of the muscles (or fascia) on the bottom of your foot, just in front of your heel. The pain can be located throughout most of the sole of your foot and make getting around painful, if not impossible.

Most of the time the cause is overuse that occurs with running, hiking, etc. Sometimes a bone spur causes the pain, and it's only diagnosed with an x-ray. Plantar fasciitis pain is usually worse from pressure (including standing on it), and oddly enough is excruciatingly painful on your first step out of bed. Padded insoles can help, but often athletes are frustrated by having to stop their workouts due to pain.

Electro-Auricular: I Hear It's All in the Ear

Believe it or not, one of my favorite treatments for plantar fasciitis involves the ear. Indeed, the Chinese, Egyptians, and Romans treated many parts of the body by stimulating acu-points in the ear.

A French neurologist named Dr. Paul Nogier began observing successful treatments of sciatica using ear acupuncture in his hometown of Lyon. He began to do more studies and experiments until he finally developed an electro-auricular non-needle acupuncture device. When it comes to treating plantar fasciitis, hikers and dancers who once suffered from the condition are now up and around and can attest to its effectiveness.

From your ear, I hear, you can treat it all!

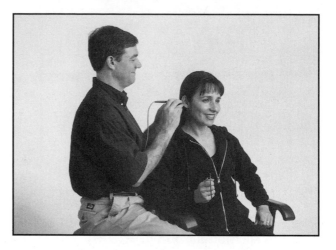

The tip of a blunt probe rests against the ear acu-point that corresponds to the area of your condition. A mild electrical current (which you don't even feel) passes into the point to promote healing.

Relieving plantar fasciitis.

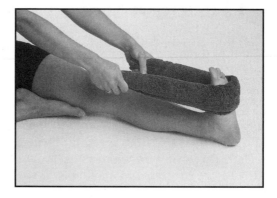

While your leg is outstretched, wrap a towel around the top part of the foot. Breathe deeply as you pull straight back with even tension. Stretch for approximately 3 seconds at a time, pointing your foot between 6 and 10 repetitions. Repeat one or two times per day to relax tight tendons and get off on the right foot.

Relieving plantar fasciitis.

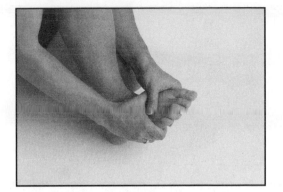

An alternate stretch for plantar fasciitis in case a towel is not handy or you want to find out which works better for you is to kneel down and grasp the front third of your feet securely in your palms. Follow the same strech outlined above with short periods of pulling back and more repetitions. This will help prevent the muscle from locking out and steadily decrease your pain.

That takes you through some of the most common conditions where pain is the reason you walk into my office. I encourage you to use the stretches and acupressure techniques that you read about earlier in this book. These would be the exercises I'd advise you to do. Talk it over with your physician and acu-pro to get his or her input. From here, we're headed for trouble, so buckle up: It's the chapter on accidents and injuries.

The Least You Need to Know

➤ Drink a glass or two of water after an acute back injury to wash out pain-causing lactic acid.

➤ Oriental Medicine and stretching are an effective back-care team.

➤ Nagging sciatic nerve pain can be shut down with acupuncture and deep pressure on acu-points.

➤ Mobilizing the kneecap keeps it loose and limber.

➤ Electro-auricular acupuncture is a non-needle solution for painful plantar fasciitis.

Chapter 10

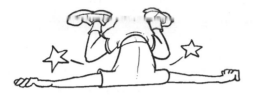

Injuries—Taking the Ouch out of the Oops!

In This Chapter

➤ Stop the painful backlash of whiplash

➤ What to do after the fall

➤ Sprained ankles from sports injuries take a hike

➤ Learn to avoid injury in the workplace

Ever since we were kids, someone has been yelling "Watch out!" and then "Too late!" We're always getting banged up at home, in our car, at work, and especially when we're out for some fun. When was the last time you heard "Oops!," followed by a loud crash?

In this chapter, you'll see how oriental medicine can help speed up the healing process from life's little injuries. We'll also discuss how to protect yourself as you return to normal activity after an injury, and how to play it safe at work by establishing healthy work habits and using ergonomics. So look both ways and slip on over to the next page.

Motor Vehicle Accidents: Putting the Brakes on Pain

Without question, automobiles have given us a great deal of freedom. On the other hand, they are perhaps the single greatest cause of injuries in the nation. According to the National Highway Traffic Safety Administration, motor vehicle accidents (MVA) are the leading cause of death for people 5–29 years of age. In 1997, the National Safety Council reported a person was injured in an MVA every 14 seconds, for a whopping 2.3 million injuries per year. In 1998, 53,000 bicyclists and 69,000 pedestrians were injured in MVAs.

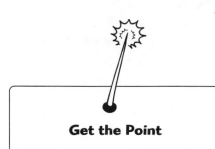

Get the Point

Watch where you step! According to the National Safety Council, accidents rank as the fourth leading cause of death worldwide behind heart disease, cancer, and strokes.

End the Backlash of Whiplash

Whiplash is the common name for an injury that affects the neck and upper back. This injury normally occurs in an MVA when your auto hits something, you suddenly stop with a rapid flexion (head and neck launch forward), followed by a rapid extension (head snaps back), or vice versa.

The damage from whiplash is often widespread throughout the neck and upper back. Symptoms range from a dull ache with stiffness to severe pain and frozen neck. Whiplash is often a difficult condition to treat, but I have found that Oriental Medicine with its bag of tools—including acupuncture, moxibustion, herbs, Tui-Na, and acupressure—can speed up recovery considerably.

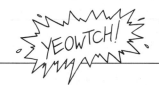

Harm Alarm

Avoid re-injury by knowing where you are in the stages of healing:

➤ Stage 1—No symptoms with minimal activities

➤ Stage 2—No symptoms with normal work or home activities

➤ Stage 3—No symptoms with extra activities such as sports or strenuous work

Match your activities with the stage. Be patient so you don't do too much too fast.

If you get whiplash, apply ice for the first 48 hours, along with massage and acupressure. You can start applying heat after about the first week. Take a look at Chapter 2, "What to Expect on Your First Visit—Does It Hurt?" for some of the acu-points to lessen the pain and speed up the gain.

The two most common muscles affected by whiplash are the scalenes—both the anterior (located at the front of neck) and posterior (located at the back of neck). Stretching both will help your neck muscles do their job of holding your head up high.

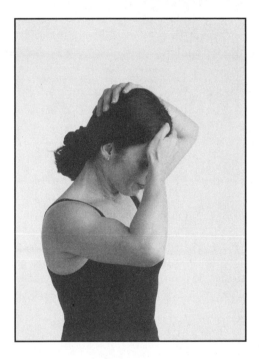

Stretching your neck muscles.

Place one hand on your forehead and the other wraps the back of your head. Both hands stabilize your injured neck while you perform the exercise. Take a deep breath in and gently stretch your head forward for a 2–3 second count as you exhale. Remember to go easy and stop if you experience too much discomfort. You are attempting to rehabilitate injured muscles, and that requires time and patience. Repeat the exercise for three to six repetitions in the beginning, increasing the number of repetitions as you gain strength and flexibility. Alternate this exercise with the anterior scalene (see the next figure).

Stretching your neck muscles.

Place your hands in the same position on the forehead, back of the head positions outlined in the preceding figure. This time you will be tilting your head back to strengthen and stretch the anterior scalenes, which are the paired muscle group that holds up your head along with the posterior scalenes. Repeat the same gentle stretch as outlined previously and be careful not to overdo it. Give yourself time to heal. This exercise will isolate the anterior scalenes that are often weak following an accident, and prevent full recovery.

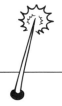

Get the Point

Your acu-pro wants to know just how bad your injury is. Here's a numbering system your professional may use in order to know how much you hurt:

➤ 0—No pain, no problem

➤ 1—25 percent reduction in work and lifestyle due to injury

➤ 2—50 percent reduction in work and lifestyle.

➤ 3—75 percent impaired by injury

➤ 4—100 percent disability, cannot perform work or normal daily activities at all

Slips and Falls: Stop Pain from Falling Through the Cracks

Now that you know how dangerous it is on the road, is it safe to stay home? Well, 40 percent of all musculoskeletal injuries occur around the house. The National Safety Council says the total cost of home injuries in 1997 was $99.9 billion. Whether you slip in the tub, slide on ice, or trip over marbles left on the floor, your first reaction is to put your hand out to catch yourself. This maneuver usually results in at least a wrist sprain.

Oriental medicine is teaming with techniques to treat all kinds of musculoskeletal home injuries, including those that affect your wrist. Expect to use acupuncture to ease your pain, herbs for both topical and internal healing, and medical Qi Gong to keep the joints open and moving.

In the meantime, here are some tips to help prevent at-home injuries in the future:

➤ Walk through every room in your house and look for risks of falls, especially where older people live or visit.

➤ Install smoke detectors and fire extinguishers.

➤ Develop a fire escape plan.

➤ Post emergency numbers (police, fire, and ambulance) where everyone can find them in a hurry.

➤ Eliminate choking or suffocating hazards for small children.

➤ Ensure your children have a lead-free environment.

If you do fall and injure your wrist, here are a few exercises that will help speed your recovery.

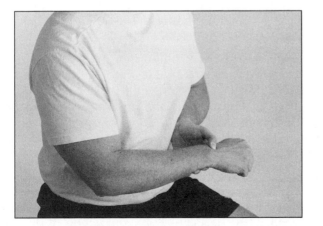

Aiding recovery of a wrist injury.

Place your injured wrist in the fingers of the other hand. This will help you control your pressure. Press firmly for one minute into TH-5 (Outer Gate), located in the middle of your arm three fingers from the wrist crease, and TH-4 (Pool of Yang), which is in the hollow place between the tendons of the top of your wrist. Keep breathing while you press on the exhale. Be gentle; you may need to use ice on swollen wrists until the circulation of qi and blood are well on their way.

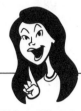

Wise Words

Barefoot doctors in China serve the rural villages that do not have access to trained physicians or hospitals. They usually have the equivalent of a high school diploma plus additional medical training, and are relied upon to treat a wide variety of conditions and injuries. They are recognized as a medical professional similar to our own community paramedics. Traditionally they worked in the community alongside other farmers in the rice patty fields, rolling up their pant legs and going barefoot. Hence the name barefoot doctor.

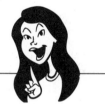

Wise Words

A standard acronym for care following an acute traumatic injury is RICE. R is for Rest; do not use the affected area. I is for Ice; apply ice packs to reduce swelling. C is for Compression; use a compression bandage to control swelling. And E is for Elevation; keep the injured area raised to avoid increasing swelling and pain.

Sports—No Guts, No Glory

I love to go out and have a great time playing sports. It builds teamwork and helps me maintain a competitive edge. Unfortunately, some of the outings result in injuries. Twenty percent of all musculoskeletal injuries in this country occur during sporting activities or on playgrounds, according to the American Academy of Orthopedic Physicians.

One of the most common sports-related injuries is the sprained ankle, whether it's turning quickly during a soccer match or running on a basketball court. Most of the time the ankle rolls to the outside, pulling the thick ligaments that hold the bones of the ankle together just a little bit too long. The result is pain, swelling, and weakness. Your acu-pro can help you quite a bit with faster healing of ligaments and tendons.

Oriental medicine has an entire branch of treatments call *Dit-Da* or hit medicine (trauma medicine). When I studied this specialty, I was amazed by all the special herbal mixtures, herbal washes, poultices, acupuncture, and massage techniques that were used to speed up the healing of traumatic musculoskeletal injuries.

The most dangerous time is when the swelling goes down, and you're back on your feet. Your ligaments have been stretched out and will not go back to their original size. Your best chance at avoiding re-injury is to strengthen the muscles in the lower leg and ankle. Work with your acu-pro and your regular doc to come up with safe, effective, muscle-building leg exercises.

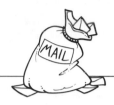

Mailbag

Sandy came limping into my office complaining of a sprained ankle that had just not gotten any better over the past month. She was a college professor who had been checked out by her physician for fractures, but did not want to take medications because they had a history of bothering her stomach. She was nearing the end of her term and had a lot of lecturing and running around to do. Except now she wasn't running much at all. She had painful swelling on the outside of her ankle that would increase with prolonged standing or walking. I began by using a specialty in Oriental Medicine called Dit-Da or hit medicine. This is often used following traumatic injuries and is composed of multiple techniques to facilitate rapid healing. With Sandy I used acupuncture, both needle and biomagnetic, Tui-Na massage, and external Chinese herbs to soak her foot in. Within the first two visits she found a marked change in swelling and pain. By the end of the second week I showed her how to do some stretching and strengthening exercises. I saw her twice a week for three weeks and then once a week for two more weeks. She then added home biomagnetic acupuncture to her treatments and cut back her visits to every other week for two more visits. She was able to do everything she needed to do and learned to care for her ankle at the same time.

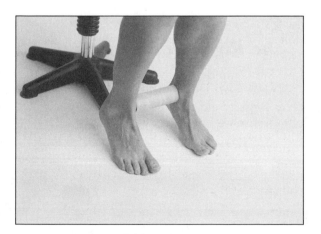

Strengthening your lower leg and ankle muscles.

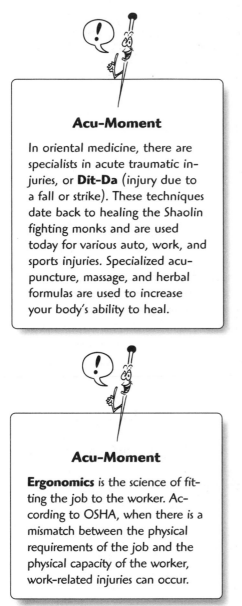

With your feet flat on the floor, place a cardboard tube (like a toilet or paper towel tube) between your ankles. Without dropping the tube, lift up your heels and toes and press the balls of your feet into the floor. This will stretch and strengthen the muscles in the outside of your ankle and leg, leaving your legs stronger and less likely to sprain again.

Work: Beyond the Job Description

Hi ho, hi ho, it's off to work we go. Unfortunately, some of us come back from work feeling worse than others do. The National Safety Council estimates that a disabling injury occurred every eight seconds in 1998 for a staggering 3.8 million injuries in that year alone. The total price tag for these injuries was $125.1 billion!

The Occupational Safety and Health Administration (OSHA) proposed new federal guidelines for *ergonomic* standards. This move is designed to protect an estimated 27 million American workers from musculoskeletal disorders (MSDs) caused from repetitive motion, force, awkward positions, and overexertions of muscles.

Some of the most common MSDs involve injuring the wrists and back (see Chapter 9, "Pain Below the Belt"). What can be done to prevent these injuries from messing up your workplace? Ergonomics.

Ergonomics—Getting the Right Position

Many employers have developed ergonomic programs to protect their workers and prevent MSDs. Check with your Human Resources Department at work to see what's available for you. Until then, look at these commonsense solutions:

➤ Reduce repeated motions and forceful hand exertions.

➤ Reduce vibration.

➤ Rely on equipment, not your back.

➤ Take mini-breaks to allow muscles to recover.

Acu-Moment

In oriental medicine, there are specialists in acute traumatic injuries, or **Dit-Da** (injury due to a fall or strike). These techniques date back to healing the Shaolin fighting monks and are used today for various auto, work, and sports injuries. Specialized acupuncture, massage, and herbal formulas are used to increase your body's ability to heal.

Acu-Moment

Ergonomics is the science of fitting the job to the worker. According to OSHA, when there is a mismatch between the physical requirements of the job and the physical capacity of the worker, work-related injuries can occur.

➤ Find different options for prolonged bending or working above shoulder height.

➤ Use a different set of muscles by varying tasks.

➤ Adjust the height of your workstation. Your upper arm and forearm should form a right angle when hands are placed on a keyboard or work surface.

➤ Adjust your computer screen so it's no higher than eye level.

➤ Place your computer monitor 18–30 inches from your eyes and place paperwork at the same height on the side of your dominant eye to avoid excess neck and shoulder strain.

This chapter highlights your acu-pro as a professional to call when you have the misfortune of being in the wrong place at the wrong time. Many of the tips to reduce the chance of injuries in your life are common sense, but are not necessarily followed. Remember that your acu-pro can substantially reduce the recovery time from an injury and assist you in a full recovery so you do not experience lingering symptoms—the old "that's my football injury when I was in high school" line. I often work in concert with the patient's physician and physical therapist during the rehabilitation phase; remember to add your acu-pro to your team. Looking ahead at the next chapter, it's time for some of the nerve-related conditions to which Oriental Medicine may offer a helping hand.

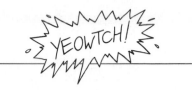

Harm Alarm

If the soda machine takes your money, just walk away. The *Journal of the American Medical Association* documented the injuries sustained by people who were trying to get a soda can out of a machine. The statistics are scary: 15 people were crushed, 3 died, and 12 were hospitalized. A fully loaded machine weights over 1,000 pounds, and the sodas are located in the top part of the machine, making the machine top-heavy and easy to tip over.

The Least You Need to Know

➤ Dit-Da uses specialized techniques of Oriental Medicine to treat acute traumatic musculoskeletal injuries.

➤ Stretching the anterior and posterior scalene muscles of your neck can end whiplash pain and stiffness.

➤ After an injury, use RICE: Rest, Ice, Compression, and Elevation.

➤ Reduce risks of home injury by developing fire escape and fall prevention plans.

➤ Follow the ergonomic checklist for a safer workplace.

Chapter 11

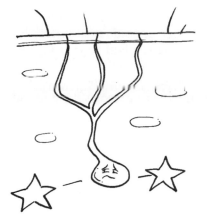

Nervous About Nerve Pain?

In This Chapter

➤ Beat Bell's palsy with Oriental Medicine

➤ Aid for limping limbs of multiple sclerosis

➤ Stop the sting of shingles

➤ Stroke recovery with acu-points

➤ Trim the pain of trigeminal neuralgia

Nerves carry signals constantly throughout a vast interlocking network of fibers in our body; like a great phone system, when it's working well, all the messages get through with precision and clarity. But what happens if the system has a few malfunctions? What if there are some missed connections, or the switch gets stuck in the "on" position? The short answer is that you experience pain—sometimes excruciating pain.

This chapter will help you check out your wiring and see how Oriental Medicine deals with some potentially devastating conditions such as Bell's palsy, multiple sclerosis, and strokes. We also will look at the nerve pains of shingles and trigeminal neuralgia. All of these conditions involve damage to the nervous system.

There's no need to be nervous now. Keep reading to discover the very real help that is available for you.

Bell's Palsy: For a Winning Smile

Imagine waking up in the morning and not being able to smile on one side of your face. Even if you weren't a morning person, you'd notice one side of your face is

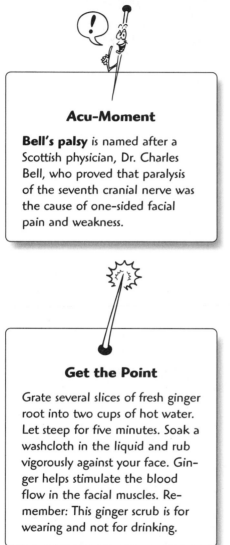

drooping. Your first thought might be that you've had a stroke, but it's probably *Bell's palsy*, a condition that affects a facial nerve on the entire side of your face. Although a stroke can affect just one side, it usually involves the whole side of the body, including the muscles of the leg and arm, beginning below the eye.

From a conventional standpoint, no one knows what causes Bell's palsy, but according to Oriental Medicine, a cold wind seems to be the cruel culprit. And, interestingly enough, exposure to severe cold often occurs before the onset of the condition. I had a patient who was a chef working in a hot kitchen. He took out the trash on a severely cold and windy night. By the time he returned, he felt tingling sensations on one side of his face, and by the next morning he had the characteristic drooping of his eyes, forehead, and mouth.

No matter the cause, time can be a healer for some of these cases while other victims may retain a degree of drooping. Don't dismay— help is on the way!

Acu-points can speed up the healing process and bring rapid results. Points used include LI-19 (Grain Seam), GB-14 (Yang White), and GB-20 (Pool of Wind). (See Chapter 7, "Pain from the Neck Up," for the location of point GB-20, and the following figure for the rest.) Press firmly on the points for one to two minutes, alternating with rubbing and kneading techniques.

Hot facial compresses (such as the one recommended in the preceding sidebar), magnets, and internal herbs are also recommended. Your acupuncturist will provide treatment not only to the affected side of the face, but also to acu-points known to have an effect on this region, as well as those that fit the overall Oriental Medical view of the patient. Electro acupuncture is commonly used for this condition because of its ability to stimulate the Qi channels more than regular needle acupuncture alone. I've had great success bringing back a winning smile to patients with Bell's palsy, so seek help from your local acu-pro if you suffer from this condition.

Acu-Moment

Bell's palsy is named after a Scottish physician, Dr. Charles Bell, who proved that paralysis of the seventh cranial nerve was the cause of one-sided facial pain and weakness.

Get the Point

Grate several slices of fresh ginger root into two cups of hot water. Let steep for five minutes. Soak a washcloth in the liquid and rub vigorously against your face. Ginger helps stimulate the blood flow in the facial muscles. Remember: This ginger scrub is for wearing and not for drinking.

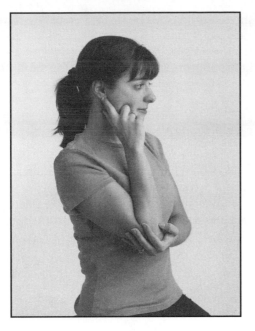

Using acupressure to relieve Bell's palsy.

Find the soft, tender spot located behind the middle of your ear lobe in between your jawbone and the mastoid process that is the bone behind the ear. This is a main acu-point for Bell's palsy, TH-17 (Shielding Wind). Apply gentle but firm pressure with your index finger for one to two minutes while breathing deeply. Other influential acu-points include SI-19 (Palace of Hearing) in front of the ear, and GB-14 (Yang White), located one finger width above the middle of the eyebrow. Use strong pressing and rubbing techniques for one to two minutes, repeating two or three times per day.

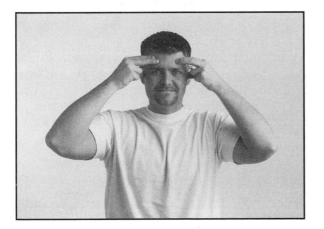

Using acupressure to relieve Bell's palsy.

Locate SI-19 (Palace of Hearing), which is in the middle of the depression formed directly in front of the ear when your mouth is open, and GB-14 (Yang White), located one finger directly above the center of your eyebrow. These points can be pressed one

105

at a time or together. The picture shows both points being stimulated by resting your index and ring fingers on GB-14 and your thumb on SI-19. Press firmly into the points for five to eight seconds and/or rub them in a circular pattern for twenty to thirty seconds. I normally recommend doing acupressure on both sides of the face in order to help the overworked side as well.

Multiple Sclerosis: A Nervous Situation

About 350,000 people in the United States have been diagnosed with MS, with approximately 200 new cases every week. Women are affected twice as often as men. Caucasians are diagnosed more frequently than African Americans or Asians. "Heavy," "stiff," "numb," and "tingling" are words that patients with multiple sclerosis often use to describe the way their muscles feel, especially the muscles in their legs.

The cause of this potentially debilitating condition is unknown, at least from a Western medical perspective. The possible causes for MS range from genetics and auto-immune disorders (the body fights against itself) to exposure to environmental factors like a virus or bacteria.

Oriental Medicine traces a similar feeling of heaviness to excessive dampness in the Qi channels.

We do know that with MS, the protective coating around nerve cells (myelin) is slowly destroyed, which interrupts or delays the transmission of nerve signals. A "short circuit" in your body's wires or nerves is what you end up with in MS—sometimes on, sometimes off. It can be maddening.

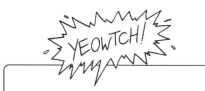

Harm Alarm

Watch how much fat you eat and what type of fat it is. The Swank Diet, named after Dr. Roy Swank, reveals that MS only occurs in countries where saturated animal fats like butter, milk, and cheese are consumed in large quantities. It's observed that high-unsaturated fats (fish oil, olive oils) are eaten in countries where MS is virtually absent.

Lighten the Load of Your Legs with Acupuncture

Acupuncture can be very effective during the early stages of MS. The techniques of needle or electro-acupuncture, along with herbal medicine, can be of considerable help in slowing down and even greatly alleviating the heavy, numb feelings in your limbs. It can be a real relief. The longer you wait for treatment, the more difficult it becomes to turn the tide of healing your way.

In addition to acupuncture and herbal therapy, some patients with MS have found relief through the practice of apitherapy; honeybee venom is injected by a hypodermic needle or by holding a honeybee and letting it sting the patient. The venom apparently acts like an anti-inflammatory and reduces leg fatigue, cramping, and spasms.

Shingles: Not Just on Your Roof

Most of us have had chicken pox in our lives. Shingles are caused from the same virus, *Varicella zoster,* also known as herpes zoster. Once you've had chicken pox, this virus may lie dormant in your body until a serious illness, emotional trauma, or prolonged stress weakens your immune system. Each year, 850,000 Americans are diagnosed with shingles.

The first sign of shingles may be chills or fever, followed by an eruption of tiny blisters that may be extremely painful and sensitive to the touch—so sensitive that something as light as a bedsheet may feel unbearable to the skin. These blisters form crusty scabs that look like roof shingles and eventually fall off. For some, this is the end of the bout, but for about 20 percent of all patients, the pain travels through the nerves. This condition is called post-zoster pain, which is a quite painful condition that can continue for a long time, especially in those with immune deficiencies.

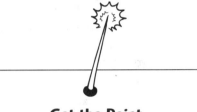

I have seen patients with severe pain spreading across their ribs, back, and belly experience great relief from acupuncture treatment. If you have shingles and visit an acupuncturist, expect the practitioner to use needle or electroneedle acupuncture around the nerves that are inflamed. So if he or she begins in the back and follows the ribs around to your chest, you'll have a lovely pattern of acupuncture needles following the nerve pathways. In my experience, you can expect to feel some relief after a couple of treatments with a cumulative effect as more sessions are given. Home care is limited for this condition outside of herbal medicine and biomagnetic treatments that reinforce your acu-pro's sessions.

For people with immune deficiencies, post-zoster pain can be severely painful. There is no known cure for this condition, and I believe that acupuncture offers real solutions for a pain that definitely gets under your skin.

Get the Point

Stay as calm and relaxed as possible and you'll do a great deal to help alleviate symptoms of MS. When stress begins to knock at your door, close your eyes, breathe in deeply through your nose, and say silently to yourself, "I am ...." Breathe out through your mouth and say to yourself, "... healthy and relaxed." Remember a time when you were at peace with yourself and the world. Try 10 slow, deep breaths to keep stress at bay. Keep breathing!

Stroke: A One-Sided Issue

Oriental medicine offers highly effective treatment options for victims of strokes. "Stroke" is the common name for a cerebrovascular accident (CVA), which damages the brain by limiting the blood supply. Stroke affects 500,000 people each year, is the third-leading cause of death in the United States each year, and is the leading cause of adult disability.

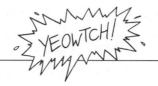

Harm Alarm

A stroke is a medical emergency and has a critical window of time when you need to recognize the warning signs and seek treatment. The side and portion of the brain affected will determine the exact symptoms.

➤ Sudden onset of numbness

➤ Weakness or clumsiness in one or both sides

➤ Double vision

➤ Severe dizziness or unsteadiness

➤ Loss of vision in one or both eyes

➤ Loss of speech or slurred speech

➤ Sudden, severe headache

The person having the stroke often denies the obvious symptoms. If you suspect you or someone else is having a stroke, seek emergency care immediately.

Your heart delivers much-needed blood to your brain through several large arteries and smaller blood vessels. Blood feeds your brain nutrients and oxygen. In a stroke, a blood clot or ruptured blood vessel in or near the brain interrupts the blood supply. The symptoms of a stroke reflect the location of the area of the brain that's being starved of blood.

Stroke: Are You at Risk?

There are several known risk factors when it comes to stroke, including

➤ **Age.** Two-thirds of all strokes affect individuals over 65.

➤ **High blood pressure.** Nearly 70 percent of stroke victims have high blood pressure.

➤ **Irregular heartbeat.** Fifteen percent of stroke patients have atrial fibrillation.

➤ **Atherosclerosis.** A buildup of fatty plaque in the arteries causes them to harden and is the leading cause of stroke and heart attacks.

➤ **Smoking.** This activity increases the buildup of cholesterol in the arteries.

➤ **Diabetes.** Diabetes prevents the body from processing fats and sugars efficiently and increases risk of both stroke and heart disease.

➤ **Race.** African-Americans have one of the highest rates of stroke in the world.

➤ **Birth control history.** Use of birth control pills combined with smoking or other risk factors can increase the rate of strokes even in young women.

The Oriental View

In China and in a growing number of countries, oriental medicine is used to treat stroke in combination with conventional medications and physical and occupational therapy. One study reviewed in the *American Journal of Acupuncture* (Vol. 21, Nov. 2, 1993) stated that 87.5 percent of patients had good response to acupuncture designed to reduce arm/leg paralysis. The results were not affected by how long it had been since the stroke. It did matter, however, how much of the brain was damaged during the stroke. (Check with your physician. A CAT scan to check brain damage is a typical diagnostic procedure in cases of stroke.)

Your acu-pro will first determine the kind of stroke you've had in oriental medical terms. Remember our discussion of internal versus external in Chapter 6, "How You Get Sick—The Good, the Bad, and the Ugly." An internal stroke may cause a loss of speech, coma, or paralysis of one side of the body known in Western terms as hemiplegia. With external strokes, patients would experience only the paralysis or numbness on one side.

Treatment methods depend on which of two symptoms present themselves: tense or loose. In a tense stroke, the hands and mouth are clenched because the muscles are tight. In this case, we want to create strong circulation to relax the muscles and increase blood and qi flow. In a loose stroke, limbs are relaxed, eyes are closed, and overall energy is weak and low.

The stronger techniques of acupuncture, such as electro-acupuncture, cupping, and firm acupressure, are reserved for the tense stroke, while milder techniques are used for the loose stroke. Your acu-pro may also use standard stroke treatments such as scalp acupuncture to help jump-start your brain, laser acupuncture, and herbal medicine. Acupressure techniques are similar to those used for MS in the previous section. The degree of force depends on whether the muscles are tense or loose.

> **YEOWTCH!**
>
> **Harm Alarm**
>
> Make sure your acu-pro knows your blood pressure level. If your blood pressure is above 200/120, the practitioner should avoid using strong needle stimulation and should perform electro-acupuncture with great caution. Have your acu-pro check your blood pressure to make sure these helpful techniques are right for you.

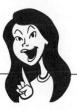

Wise Words

Bad habits can wear you down over time, and according to traditional oriental medicine, make you more susceptible to stroke. Try to avoid or limit the following:

➤ Overwork

➤ Physical and emotional stress

➤ Inadequate rest

➤ Excess sexual activity

➤ Poor diet

Creating balance in your life can lessen your risk for strokes.

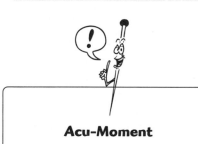

Acu-Moment

Aretaeous described **trigeminal neuralgia** in the first century A.D. Early treatments included bloodletting, along with bandages coated with poison such as arsenic, mercury, hemlock, and cobra and bee venoms. An eighteenth-century French surgeon, Nicolaus Andre, gave it the name "tic douloureux," which means "painful spasm."

Trigeminal Neuralgia: Facing Your Pain

There are three facial nerve branches involved in the condition known as *trigeminal neuralgia,* or tic douloureux. It's as if the pain switch gets left on when it comes to the ophthalmic area, which runs along the forehead, eye, or nose. The areas involved include the maxillary area, which affects your upper teeth, cheek, and lower eyelid, and the mandibular area, which encompasses the lower teeth, lip, and jaw.

Which area is painful to you depends on which of the three nerve branches has become damaged. The pain is described by many as the most terrible pain known to humankind. This pain is on one side of your face and is experienced as short bursts of electrical shocks. The shocks may only last for a few seconds, but a series of attacks can repeat within a minute, making it difficult to do the simplest things. Often, a simple touch to one area of the face can trigger an attack. Eating, washing, shaving, and even applying makeup can be tricky propositions.

What causes trigeminal nerve pain? Here are a few possibilities:

➤ Pressure of blood vessel on trigeminal nerve root

➤ Protective coating of nerve destroyed (as in multiple sclerosis)

➤ Pressure of tumor on trigeminal nerve (rare)

➤ Damage to nerve by dental or surgical procedures

➤ Unknown—many cases have no clear cause

Help with Acupuncture

Acupuncture may offer some help to those suffering from trigeminal neuralgia. Unlike other conditions where a splint or bandage tells everyone you're hurting, this condition shows no obvious outward signs except the wince of your face when the pain hits. Wind (Shooting Pains) is traditionally how trigeminal neuralgia is characterized in Oriental Medicine. Needle, ear, or electro-auricular (see Chapter 9, "Pain Below the Belt," on plantar fasciitis) have been the ways I've dealt successfully with giving relief. There are no guarantees with medicine, and this condition is no exception. I believe that acupuncture is worth pursuing as a viable treatment option.

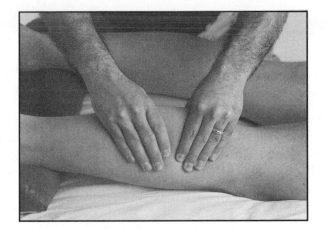

Relieving trigeminal nerve pain.

To perform this technique, you will need someone to help administer the acupressure to the stroke patient. Have him or her go to the side affected by the stroke. Use kneading and grasping techniques combined with palm pressure on the large flat muscles on the inside and outside of the arms and legs. Remember to grasp the muscles and hold for about five seconds. Press them firmly with your palm. Use pressure to fit the particular condition. You may repeat this procedure two to three times throughout the day using gentle yet firm direct pressure.

The neurological conditions that we've just reviewed lend themselves to a limited amount of self-care at first. As your condition improves there are many of the acupressure techniques that will be valuable to your continued recovery. For our next chapter, take a deep breath in; we're about to go into your respiration. So breath easy and follow me.

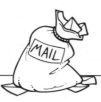

Mailbag

Donna was about to lose her mind. Not only was she trying to hold down a job in which she was often out on a sick day, she could barely function at home with her family due to the debilitating pain of trigeminal neuralgia. Her pain began following a dental procedure, and a series of medications and other procedures had not been able to lessen her daily discomfort. She began to cry as she related the pain she faced during the course of a normal day, and how she felt bad that her children had to watch her suffer. She was unable to participate in life as she wanted to and had already lost hope when she turned the handle and entered my office. A friend had recommended that she try acupuncture to find out if it could help, even just a little. Donna experienced most of her pain along the nerve pathway beside her nose. Terrible shooting pains would take her breath away. We tried needle acupuncture at first, but did not have any change in her condition by the fourth treatment, so I decided to use electro-auricular acupuncture, a non-needle therapy that treats the whole body through the acu-points located in the ear. I again saw her crying, but this time she informed me it was due to the pain in her face diminishing for the first time in over one year! We continued this treatment, which brought greater reduction of pain and more time was put between treatments until I have not needed to see her for several months. She has begun to laugh again, a luxury when it used to trigger pain, and is living a full and happy life with her family.

The Least You Need to Know

➤ Acu-points can perk up your smile if you've got Bell's palsy.

➤ The heavy limbs of MS are lightened by oriental medicine.

➤ Acupuncture short-circuits the shooting pains of shingles.

➤ Overwork, stress, poor diet, excessive sex, and inadequate rest are Oriental Medical risk factors for stroke.

Part 3

Respiration, Perspiration, and Menstruation

Take a deep breath and hang on through a series of chapters dealing with life's challenges that can be alleviated by oriental medicine. Brace yourself for the relief of many common breathing ailments such as allergies, asthma, and the common cold. Worn-out parents take special note of the tips for ending some of your worst nightmares: colic, coughs, ear infections, and, yes … diarrhea (in the clinic we call it the gift that keeps on giving!). Various types of cancer treatments using oriental medicine are outlined in this part of the book, giving patients options during perhaps the most challenging time in their lives. Finally, we take a look at many of the oriental solutions that are available to balance hormones and monthly cycles for women who are tired of suffering on a regular basis. Keep turning these pages and soak up the knowledge that has been passed down through the ages for you to use.

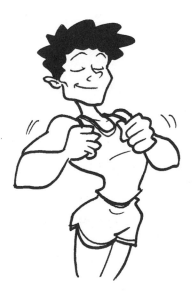

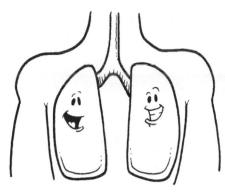

Chapter 12

Respiration—
A Breath of
Fresh Air

In This Chapter

➤ Keys to springing yourself from perennial allergy prison

➤ Oriental medicine helps asthma sufferers breathe with confidence

➤ Break up bronchitis

Breathing is mostly taken for granted … until we have to struggle to take a good deep breath. Whether your nose is stuffed up or your lungs feel tight, it becomes an obsession to breath, especially when you can't!

In this chapter, we give you hope of treating your awful allergies and asthma. Oriental Medicine once more comes to the rescue in the case of bronchitis. We'll take a look at the issues of allergies, their treatment, and prevention. Asthma and bronchitis sufferers will get tips on self-care techniques using acu-points and medical massage. Life can be challenging enough without struggling for each breath. Now it's time to begin your journey to better breathing.

Allergies: Aahh-Choo!

I remember having mixed emotions about the coming of spring, because I suffered from hay fever. The winter was over, the sun was out—but so were tree pollens and grasses. If you've ever had seasonal allergies (*allergic rhinitis*), you know the feeling: itchy, watery eyes, waterfalls from your running nose, irritability, fatigue, sneezing, and more sneezing. At first you might think it's a cold, but allergies do not come with a fever, and the nasal discharge is runny and clear, instead of the yellow-to-green thicker stuff that's typical of a cold.

Acu-Moment

Allergic rhinitis (hay fever) brings about reactions to airborne pollens and grasses. Symptoms occur between February and the fall. **Perennial rhinitis** is characterized by hay fever symptoms all year round. It can be triggered by environmental factors such as animal hair, food additives, feathers, or fungus.

Put a Close to the Runny Nose

Oriental medicine can offer significant relief for allergy sufferers; I got help, and so can you. The kind of traditional oriental diagnosis you have is determined by your symptoms. With allergies, your immune system is overreacting to some outside substance, and your individual characteristics will point the way for your acu-pro.

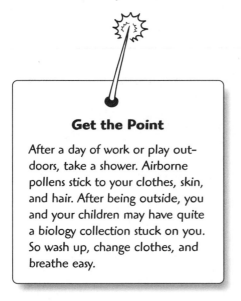

Get the Point

After a day of work or play outdoors, take a shower. Airborne pollens stick to your clothes, skin, and hair. After being outside, you and your children may have quite a biology collection stuck on you. So wash up, change clothes, and breathe easy.

One factor to consider is your general energy level. If you are tired and lethargic even before allergy season, then part of your treatment strategy will be to rebuild your energy level and improve your immune system. You'll generally feel better and have a better chance at alleviating awful allergies.

Herbal medicine is frequently used with acupuncture to alleviate sinus pressure and stop your waterfall nose. I've instructed patients to use biomagnets as a self-care home treatment in between visits. All of these techniques have worked well for relieving and sometimes completely ending chronic allergy complaints. A word of advice, though; start treatment of allergic rhinitis a few months before the allergy season hits. This will give your body a chance to change in order to lessen or eliminate the seasonal symptoms.

Acupressure: Keys to End the Sneeze

Acupressure is a great way to temporarily alleviate a runny nose. The best part is that you always have your tools at hand.

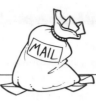

Mailbag

Jack prides himself in being fit. He is an avid runner and road cyclist who also practices daily yoga and is conscientious about his nutrition. Two years ago he came to me mortified that seasonal allergies in the spring and fall had given way to year-round sniffling and sneezing. He felt that energized, peppy demeanor start to be dulled down and he did not like it a bit. We began with acupuncture, but quickly found that the environmental influences were too strong to allow the treatments to have their desired long-lasting effect. I prescribed a custom herbal formula that took into consideration the allergy symptoms as well as his unique physical, mental, and emotional make-up. I had raw herbs ground into a powder, which was encapsulated for more convenience, taken one to three times per day. By the end of his third week he reported considerable improvement. Within two months his allergy symptoms had all but gone, and he felt much better over all—even in areas that had little to do with his chief complaint. I see Jack about once every six months to update his prescription for the change of seasons and his continually improving health.

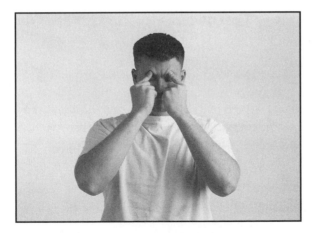

Alleviating a runny nose.

Find acu-points Yuyao (Fish Waist) located in the eyebrow directly above the pupil of the eye, and LI-20 (Welcome Fragrance) in the crease of skin beside the nostrils. Breathe slowly and deeply as you press firmly for one minute on the exhale. Stimulate one or both points at a time. Repeat three to five times, and throughout the day as needed. You may also add pressure to LI-4 (Adjoining Valleys). See Chapter 7, "Pain from the Neck Up," on wrist pain for details. Do not use this point if you are pregnant.

117

Asthma: Ease the Wheeze

Asthma affects more than 10 million Americans (3 million children and 7 million adults). Children under 16 and adults over 65 are more likely to have asthma. Hospitalizations due to this condition have increased 500 percent in the last 29 years, while the death rate in the U.S. from asthma has increased 45 percent in the past 10 years.

Asthma is a condition that blocks the flow of air into your lungs. During an asthma attack, spasms in the muscles surrounding the bronchi (small airways in the lungs) make the air passages smaller. This makes you feel like you have to fight for every breath, and most people experience symptoms such as coughing, wheezing (the raspy, sucking sound as you breathe), and a feeling of tightness in the chest. These spasms of the airways are commonly triggered by hypersensitivity to environmental factors.

Common Asthma Triggers

➤ Animal dander

➤ Dust mites

➤ Tobacco smoke

➤ Environmental pollutants

➤ Food additives (sulfites)

➤ Change in temperature

➤ Low-blood sugar

➤ Extremes of dryness or humidity

➤ Respiratory infection

➤ Chemicals

➤ Fumes

➤ Molds

➤ Feathers

➤ Anxiety

➤ Exercise

➤ Weather changes

There are several known causes of asthma, including the following:

➤ **Early-onset asthma (extrinsic)**—Begins in childhood, hereditary, often associated with eczema at birth, skin reactions to environmental triggers

➤ **Late-onset asthma (intrinsic)**—Begins during adult years, coupled with upper respiratory viral infections, no hereditary or eczema component, worse from weather changes, exercise, and emotional stress

➤ **Cardiac asthma**—Asthma symptoms, but caused by heart failure

Take a Deep Breath with Acu-Points

Oriental Medicine combines several techniques for effective treatment of asthma. The 1998 report from the National Institutes of Health states: "Acupuncture treatment for many conditions such as asthma should be a part of a comprehensive management plan."

Acupuncture or acupressure techniques are not a replacement for conventional medicine, but work well in conjunction with treatment from your doctor. I have used needle, biomagnet, and electro-auricular acupuncture to effectively treat asthma. Herbal medicine, cupping, nutritional supplementation, and medical Qi Gong are also ways to get a fresh breath with the help of Oriental Medicine. I've been pleased to assist my patients in reducing or eliminating medications and return to active, more enjoyable lives.

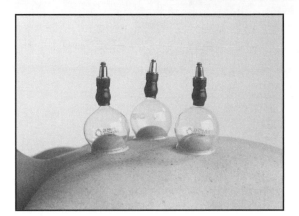

Cupping jars are placed on acu-points that help open your lungs. Your acu-pro can show you how to do this helpful technique at home.

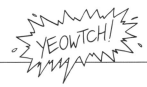

Harm Alarm

The Chinese herb Ma-Huang (also known as Ephedra) is a commonly used herb in Chinese herbal formulas for asthma and is used by conventional medicine in bronchial inhalers. It is a central nervous system stimulant and a bronchial dilator, opening bronchial passages. Unfortunately, it has been placed in many over-the-counter products like energy bars and drinks. Do not use Ma-Huang if you have anxiety, glaucoma, heart disease, high blood pressure, or insomnia, or are taking monoamine oxidase inhibitor for depression. To use this herb safely, make sure you are under the care of a qualified herbalist or physician.

You'll need a volunteer from the audience to get this useful acupressure technique. Have him or her curve his or her hands into soft round cups, then use percussion on either side of the spine with quick light tapping of the hands so a clapping sound is made. Your helper should do this for 30 seconds to one minute, while you let him or her know if the pressure feels good. This procedure will loosen up and energize the lungs. Your volunteer should avoid tapping too hard or for too long; after all, you're not a conga drum!

Loosening up the lungs.

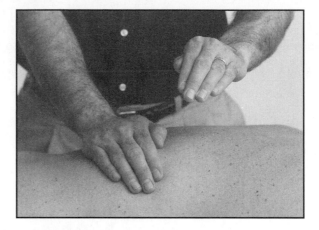

Bronchitis: Quit the Cough

Bronchitis is the inflammation or blockage of the bronchi, the breathing tubes that connect to your lungs. When they are blocked, mucus builds up and you may experience symptoms such as coughing, pain in the chest, difficulty breathing, fever, and a generally yucky, tired feeling. Acute bronchitis is caused by bacterial or viral infections, while chronic conditions result from frequent irritation of the lungs due to cigarette smoke, smog, allergies, or overexposure to cold, damp air. Mucus is not a bad thing. We need it to lubricate our lungs and filter out foreign substances like dust when they are not needed or wanted. In bronchitis, too much of a good thing causes the constant cough.

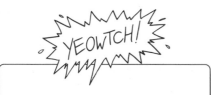

Harm Alarm

If you have a history of chronic respiratory disease or are in poor health, a cough that has gone on for too long could be a more serious condition, such as pneumonia. Consult with your physician.

Points to Cut Off the Cough

The key in relieving bronchitis is to clean away the extra mucus and open the lungs. Acu-points include Ding Chuan (Stop Wheezing), B-12 (Wind's Door), LU-1 (Central Residence), and CV-17 (Penetrating Odor). (I'm just relaying the names, folks—I didn't make them up myself!) Your acupuncturist will use these points plus others that correspond to helping your general health. Moxabustion or heat treatment may be used on your back and neck to melt the mucus, or cupping jars placed on BL-12 to dislodge mucus and open the lungs. Then, open sesame ... you enjoy better breathing. Acupressure self-care requires the right touch (see the following figures).

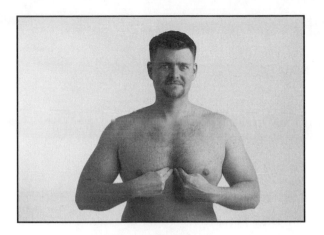

Stabilize your hands by laying them on your chest, gently at first, pressing into CV-17 (located in the middle of the sternum or breast bone between the nipples). This area may be sore from coughing, so press gently, adjusting the pressure to your comfort.

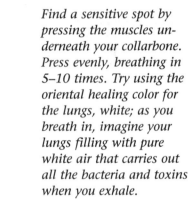

Find a sensitive spot by pressing the muscles underneath your collarbone. Press evenly, breathing in 5–10 times. Try using the oriental healing color for the lungs, white; as you breath in, imagine your lungs filling with pure white air that carries out all the bacteria and toxins when you exhale.

The same percussion techniques that were used for asthma can be used on BL-12 to fight bronchitis. Moving two fingers down from Ding Chuan and two-finger width beside your spine (see the preceding figure), put a slight curve in your hands, reach behind the top of your shoulders, and pretend you are playing the bongos. Remember to play a soothing beat. It's even better if you have a friend lend a hand to loosen the lungs.

Nutrients to Neutralize Mucus

You've spent all this time clearing your lungs of mounds of mucus. Now you need to practice avoiding sugary foods or dairy products that often gunk them up again. Even something as simple as drinking too much fruit juice translates into ingesting sugar (fructose). Try supplementing with vitamin C, which cuts the mucus without the sugar, and coenzyme Q10, which helps get rid of toxins. Black radish, mullein, chickweed, fenugreek, and gingko biloba are used to further clean mucus from your lungs. Consult an herbalist if you have any questions. He or she can guide you in your choices or create a custom prescription for your particular needs.

121

Reach over your shoulder and locate Ding Chuan, one finger width beside your spine at C-7, where your neck meets your back. Press or tap while breathing deeply for 5–10 breaths. This can be done on one point at a time or together as shown. Repeat one to three times during the day.

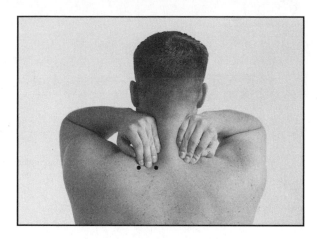

We've dealt with a few of life's aahh choos and difficulties in breathing. Never fear—hope is near for cutting back the ravages of the common cold, cough, and nasal congestion. Turn to the next chapter before you need another handkerchief.

The Least You Need to Know

➤ Oriental medicine can give relief for both allergic rhinitis (seasonal hay fever) and perennial rhinitis (year-round hay fever).

➤ Washing your hair and changing clothes after you've been outside can reduce your exposure to seasonal allergic pollens.

➤ Dust mites, tobacco smoke, and food additives are just a few of the common asthma triggers.

➤ Acupuncture techniques, including cupping, can greatly reduce worrisome asthmatic wheezing.

➤ Cutting back on sugar can help dissolve the mucus of bronchitis.

Chapter 13

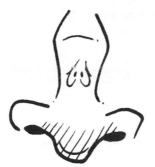

Colds—Nosing Around for Better Health

> ### In This Chapter
>
> ➤ Learn how to stop colds in their tracks
>
> ➤ Discover how Oriental Medicine cuts through your cough
>
> ➤ Acu-points to negate nasty nasal congestion
>
> ➤ Say "so long" to sinusitis

I live in New England, and it's not uncommon for me to see patients that keep passing the same cold around their families for weeks. I also meet a great number of people who experience a stuffed-up nose or have a cough from late fall until spring. They often say it's been that way every year and they're coming in for treatment because they're just tired of it.

If you're tired of your nose dripping, constantly clearing your throat, or blowing your nose, then read on. Chinese doctors have many alternatives for you, including a famous Chinese physician named Zhang Zhong Jing (c. 220 C.E.), who wrote *Discussions of Cold-Induced Diseases* for his patients who were also tired of having chronic colds and upper-respiratory problems. Read on to discover the ancient solutions for our modern colds and coughs.

Colds: Clearing a Common Condition

There are more than 100 viruses that have been identified as causing the common cold. Americans spend approximately one billion dollars a year on over-the-counter products to reduce or eliminate the all-too-familiar symptoms of body ache, congestion, headache, fever, or sneezing. On average, most of us experience two colds a year, with children having more than adults because their immune systems are still developing.

The key to beating back the virus of a cold is attacking it during the incubation period, typically from one to three days after exposure. During that time, your immune system is doing its best to fight on your behalf. If you are excessively tired, emotionally stressed, already sick, have a suppressed immune system, or are in the mid-phase of your menstrual cycle, then your immunity is fighting with one hand tied behind its proverbial back.

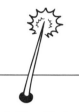

Get the Point

Try herbs to hasten the course of the cold and relieve unwanted symptoms. During the first 12–24 hours of common cold symptoms, which include body aches and nasal congestion, crush four to six white bulbs of a green scallion into a pot of boiling water. Cut up the greens from the scallions and add those as well. In addition, grate several slices of fresh ginger root and add them to the pot. Let the mixture steep for five minutes; strain off the herbs and drink a cup of the tea every two to three hours. This is an old Chinese herbal remedy I have found effective for the beginning stages of a cold.

Most colds run their course within 7 to 10 days, but if you are already sick or susceptible to upper-respiratory infections, then a cold can lead to much more serious conditions. It's best to take a stand while you can!

Oriental Medicine Calms the Cold

While there is no proven cure for the common cold, the time-tested techniques of Oriental Medicine can definitely shorten the course of your condition. Also, these methods are designed to strengthen your body's immunity to avoid secondary infections, such as bronchitis or strep, or the same cold over and over again. Because there are more than 100 viruses that cause our colds and no form of western medicine that can tame them, it makes sense to choose oriental medicine to individually diagnose and treat your cold symptoms. Rest is a common prescription—and one that's frequently ignored. Acupuncture, herbs, and cupping are also frequent fliers on this kind of trip.

Acupressure can be done on LI-20 (Welcome Fragrance), GB-20 (Wind Pond), and LI-4 (Adjoining Valleys, but remember to avoid this acu-point if you are pregnant). Apply steady, direct pressure while deeply breathing for a count of five seconds. Treatments are selected, as you've already seen throughout this text, based on a full Oriental Medical diagnosis.

Colds are considered to be external causes of illness and are generally divided into two categories: Wind Cold and Wind Heat. Wind in both cases refers to the sudden onset and external/environmental origins of the cold. Achy muscles, headache often in the back of the head, clear runny nasal discharge, chills, and a desire for warm foods and liquids characterize Wind Cold symptoms. Wind Heat Colds feel feverish, with a sore throat, a thirst with a desire for cold liquids, and a frontal headache. Depending on the pattern, a treatment plan will be given to fit your individual needs.

Cough: Expectorating to Feel Better

A cough is a sudden, explosive way to clear material from your airways, which means that having a cough is a good thing as long as it doesn't last too long.

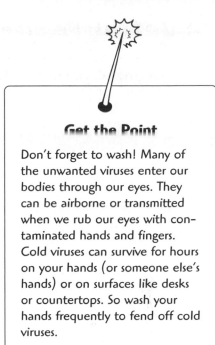

Get the Point

Don't forget to wash! Many of the unwanted viruses enter our bodies through our eyes. They can be airborne or transmitted when we rub our eyes with contaminated hands and fingers. Cold viruses can survive for hours on your hands (or someone else's hands) or on surfaces like desks or countertops. So wash your hands frequently to fend off cold viruses.

When it comes to diagnosing a cough, conventional and Oriental Medicines have much in common. Practitioners of both will ask you how long you've had it and categorize it as either acute (meaning it lasts from three to seven days) or chronic (meaning it lasts more than 10 days). They both will listen and categorize the sounds of the cough as weak, barking, loose, or rattling, each one indicating a different likely underlying cause. The time of day and the color and texture of your mucus provide further clues about what's causing you to cough.

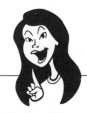

Harm Alarm

Don't stress out! Worry can actually worsen your cough. According to traditional Oriental Medicine, your emotions strongly affect the health of your lungs. Prolonged worry ties up the Qi in lungs, producing a dry, irritating cough. Anger, frustration, and resentment produce sudden coughing bouts and a dry throat, and are associated with bloating and discomfort under the ribs. So clear up whatever is bothering you and let it go, at least for the sake of your cough.

Acu-Points: Breathe a Sign of Relief

Whether your cough is characterized by wind/heat (dry cough, tickling in back of the throat) or phlegm/heat (barking cough which produces profuse yellow mucus), your acu-pro can design a treatment plan to fit your individual needs.

Treating a cough.

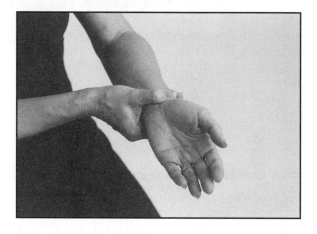

Locate LU-9 (Great Abyss) with your palm facing up; it's on your wrist crease on the same side as your thumb. Hold this point with your index finger or thumb for one to three minutes while breathing slowly and deeply. Breathe in through your nose and out your mouth. Other acu-points used for coughs include CV-17 (Penetrating Odor), LU-1 (Central Residence), and Ding Chuan (Stop Wheezing), which are all found in Chapter 12, "Respiration—A Breath of Fresh Air," in the section on bronchitis.

Nasal Congestion: Had Enough of the Stuff?

This section is for all the folks who go through their days with a stuffed-up nose; they're not actually sick, but they're not well, either. Nasal congestion can be brought on initially by a cold, but then stay around due to incomplete healing of cold symptoms or environmental allergies. Whatever the original cause, you now have a condition that makes you susceptible to even more illnesses. Oriental Medicine suggests that the nose is the gatekeeper to the lungs, which are highly sensitive to external forces. Chronic nasal congestion often opens the doors to more severe illnesses. Your acu-pro will help you untangle the causes and assist you in getting on a treatment and prevention program to keep your nasal passages open and clean.

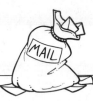

Mailbag

Bob flies across country as part of his job and has been troubled for years with chronic sinus congestion. Sometimes he gets an infection, but most of the time he's just got a nasally voice and has intermittent headaches, especially when he flies. Due to his hectic travel schedule I was only able to treat him infrequently with acupuncture. Our successes came from a combination of a customized herbal prescription, self-care acupressure at home or in the airplane, and watching the ingestion of some mucus producing foods. Today nasal congestion, or sinusitis, rarely troubles him.

Sinusitis: Inflammation in a Hidden Station

Your *sinus* cavities are open spaces located on either side of your nose. Sinuses have layers of folded-up skin (mucosa) that help regulate the pressure and keep those open spaces clean. When your immune system is low, you can get an acute attack of sinusitis (*-itis* at the end of any word means "inflammation"). Inflammation is the immune system's response to infection and is characterized by swelling, redness, heat, and pain. You may also be experiencing chronic sinusitis due to small growths (polyps) in the nose, or from allergies to environmental irritants like fumes or cigarette smoke.

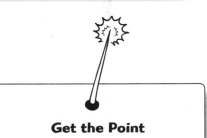

Get the Point

Your grandma was right! Drinking plenty of pure water, hot soup, and herbal teas help mucus break up and flow to relieve nasal congestion and pressure. Adding a pinch of cayenne pepper and scallions to your tea can speed up the relief.

When your sinuses are inflamed, it feels like your whole face hurts. If you tap on your forehead or just under your eyes and feel pain, you probably have an infection. You may also experience further unwanted symptoms such as low-grade fever, headache (often described as "splitting"), difficulty breathing through your nose, loss of smell, and yellow or green nasal discharge. (Yum, yum.) Unfortunately, that gunk may also be draining down your throat, creating a sore throat, nausea, snoring, or a cough.

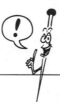

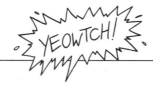

Acu-Moment

The word **sinus** is Latin meaning "curve," "fold," or "hollow." Sinus was used earlier in medieval times to mean the fold of a garment. In medicine, the term was combined to describe the sinus cavities in the human head, whose tissue looked like folded garments tucked in a hollow space.

Harm Alarm

Don't assume it's "just a cold." About 25 percent of chronic maxillary sinusitis (near your cheekbones) is caused by a dental infection. If your immune system is compromised, sinusitis can be caused from fungal infections. Check with your physician to make sure you know the root of your snout problem.

Acu-Pros Clear Your Nose

The goal is to get your sinuses to drain (remember the soggy, folded garments?). This will stop the swelling and pain, encouraging normal circulation to return, and end the thick, gunky mucus discharge. Oriental medicine does a great job at relieving both acute and chronic sinusitis. Patients are amazed at the rapid release of pressure in the sinuses that acupuncture can bring.

Herbal medicine, improved diet, and attention to potential environmental irritants can help keep your sinuses healthy once they've been cleared. Your acu-pro will determine the kind of sinusitis you have, such as wind/heat or dampness/heat, based on your symptoms. Acupuncture and acupressure create circulation of blood in the hard-to-get-to folded tissues of the sinuses. You'll enjoy letting the pressure out of your face.

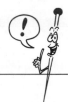

Acu-Moment

Your sinus cavities actually have many caverns and spaces. The location of your infection or inflammation could be in any of the following:

➤ Frontal sinuses, just above your eyes

➤ Ethmoid sinuses, located in your upper nose

➤ Sphenoid sinuses, found just behind the bridge of your nose

➤ Maxillary sinuses, on either side of the nose, inside the cheekbones

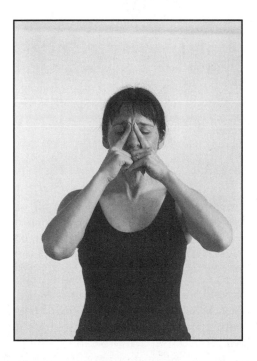

Clearing the nose.

Locate BL-2 (Gathered Bamboo) in the hollow notch at the outside end of your eyebrow. Put your hands together, steadying your thumbs under your chin and your middle fingers on your nose, as you press firmly for one minute into BL-2 with your index finger. Close your eyes and breathe deeply. Use pressure that is comfortable. Repeat several times a day to keep sinus pressure clear.

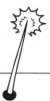

Get the Point

Be gentle with your nose! Avoid blowing your nose in a hard, forceful honk, which forces mucus back up into your sinuses and can irritate the already swollen passages. Try blowing gently out of one side at a time, or draw nasal discharge into the back of your throat and spit it out.

Bringing circulation into the sinus cavities.

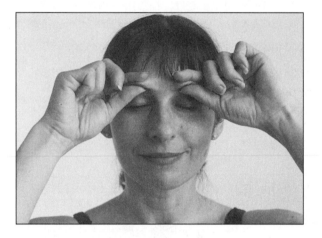

Locate Yu Yao (Fish Waist) in the center of your eyebrow. Alternate pressing the point for 30 seconds, then lifting and pinching your eyebrows to bring much-needed circulation into your sinus cavities. Remember to breathe and repeat throughout the day as needed.

The Chinese observed several thousand years ago that the nose and lungs were the outermost organs of the body and most susceptible to external forces. I believe we can all agree that colds and coughs will be with us for another few thousand years. Oriental Medicine has developed many useful strategies for reducing acute symptoms and eliminating stubborn chronic symptoms. Your acu-pro can fill you in on the options for your specific condition. Moving on, we turn our attention to our children. Turn to the next chapter and discover solutions to ease your babies' ills.

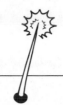

Get the Point

Try steaming your sinuses clear. Inhaling steam helps to loosen up the mucus, take the pressure off, and promote circulation and drainage. Boil a pot of water, remove it from the heat, and place a couple drops of eucalyptus or rosemary oil in the water. Put a towel over your head and lean over the pot, about six to eight inches away, but not close enough to get scalded. Breathe deeply for 5 to 10 minutes, repeating throughout the day as needed.

The Least You Need to Know

➤ Oriental Medicine helps your immune system fight back from more than 100 cold-causing viruses.

➤ Washing your hands frequently and avoiding rubbing your eyes can help keep you clear of a cold.

➤ Cutting out your cough may mean cutting back on mucus-producing foods, like dairy, sugars, or deep-fried anything.

➤ Acu-points can lessen sinus pressure and pain by opening the cavities so they can drain.

Chapter 14

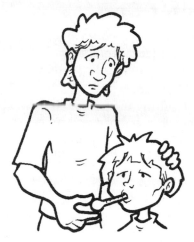

Childhood Conditions— Pass the Owner's Manual

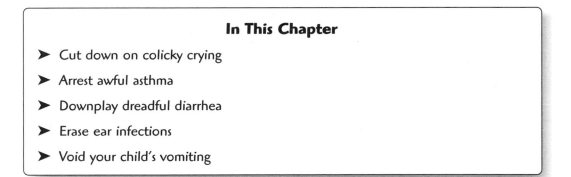

In This Chapter

➤ Cut down on colicky crying

➤ Arrest awful asthma

➤ Downplay dreadful diarrhea

➤ Erase ear infections

➤ Void your child's vomiting

Baby giggles are magical. They can melt away the day's tension and put a smile on the sourest of pusses. When you dreamed of having your baby, your visions probably included baby giggles or gazing lovingly at your toddler sleeping peacefully in your arms.

This chapter goes where no dreams dare to go ... the challenges of childhood. We'll take a look at the bubbles, burps, spurts, pops, poops, and oops that are all part of being a parent. Babies have had confused and worried parents for centuries, and Oriental Medicine has been around to help.

You'll discover that many of the techniques available can be done by you, the parents. Your acu-pro can guide and advise, but it's up to you to take action. These conditions can be frustrating to a parent who is already worn out, but the rewards of helping to heal your baby are endless. As you hold your child in one hand, use the other to turn the page and learn the power of your own healing hands.

Colic: The Bubble That Just Won't Burst

Lying down for a well-deserved sleep is just hopeful wishing if your baby is suffering from colic. Very common with infants, colic officially affects over 20 percent of all babies, although the numbers are thought to be much greater. Colic pertains to the colon (intestine), and the old word for it was the "gripe," usually pronounced *grip*.

Colic occurs when gas forms in your baby's colon, resulting in abdominal pain and spasms that we speculate feel as if the intestines are being grabbed and squeezed. To have an official diagnosis of colic, your baby must cry for three or more hours a day, on at least three days of the week, and be between the ages of three weeks and three months. Luckily, colic usually passes after three to four months, but oooh, until it does! It's tough to see your baby so unhappy.

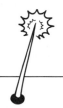

Get the Point

An old colic cure is to place a hot water bottle on your knees and lay your baby's tummy on top. Be careful it's not too hot (you may want to place a blanket or diaper between the water bottle and your baby's tummy or place the water bottle over your baby's clothes). Gently bounce your baby on your knees. Pat his or her little back as you move and sway to help the gas along the way.

Back Off the Gas: Foods to Avoid

Breast- and formula-fed babies seem to have the same amount of colic. Certainly if you are using formula, it's a good idea to switch to another brand, or try a nondairy variety to see if food intolerance is part of your baby's discomfort. You may also vary the amount you feed your baby. Overfeeding is another common cause of colic. Feeding on demand is controversial with child-rearing experts, but it's an easy experiment to try scheduled feedings of a set amount of food and see if the colic improves.

Breast-feeding mothers will also want to be careful to avoid gassing up on these foods:

➤ Cabbage   ➤ Tomatoes

➤ Broccoli   ➤ Citrus fruits

➤ Cauliflower   ➤ Garlic

- ➤ Brussels sprouts
- ➤ Coffee
- ➤ Rhubarb
- ➤ Melons

- ➤ Chocolate
- ➤ Beans
- ➤ Peaches
- ➤ Onions

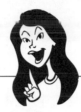

Wise Words

You can help soothe your baby's colic by giving him or her herbs with an eyedropper. For colic, use chamomile, peppermint, anise, fennel, or caraway teas. Let the tea cool and put one to two eyedroppers full of tea in the back of your baby's throat. Ask your acu-pro which tea is best for your baby's colic.

Colic Massage: Rub a Dub Dub

In many cultures, infant massage is not just a way to help heal but also a continuous way to love and bond with your new baby.

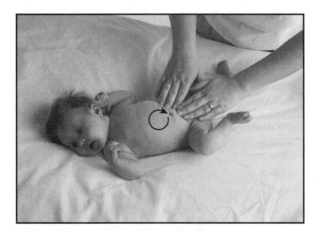

Infant massage.

Place a few drops of your favorite massage oil, or even olive oil, on your baby's tummy. Apply gentle soft pressure in a clockwise circle under the ribs and navel. This follows the path of the colon. A slow and rhythmic pattern will comfort and reassure your child. Repeat twice a day for at least one week before you judge its effects. Singing and nursery rhymes are optional and encouraged.

Again, place a few drops of your favorite massage oil or olive oil, only this time use smaller circles. Begin next to the navel and go in a clockwise direction, with smaller, gentle rhythmic motion. Continue the singing and you'll hear goo goos!

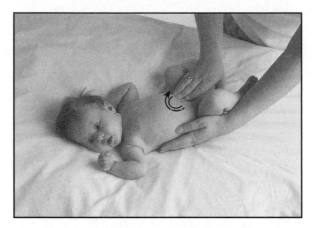

Place your thumbs beside your baby's navel, slowly and gently stretch the abdomen by moving your thumbs to the outside. Only a slight amount of pressure is needed to help your baby's digestion. Repeat 2–3 times.

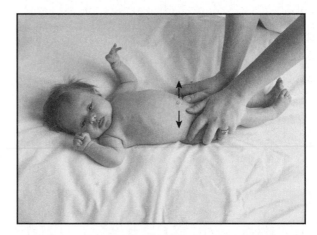

After completing a few circles as in the previous figure, move your baby's knees to his or her chest and hold for 15–30 seconds. Straighten out your baby's legs and massage them. Repeat this entire cycle two to three times daily for best results. Smile while you massage ... your baby will love it!

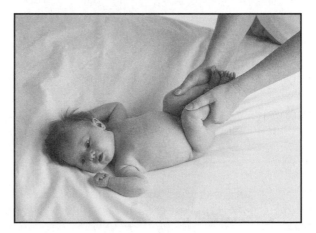

Pediatric Asthma: Silence Is Golden

Needless to say, the parental panic button goes off when your child can't breathe. This inability to breathe is caused by an overproduction of mucus and inflammation, which contracts and blocks the bronchial airways (the little tubes going into the lungs).

Asthma now affects 4.8 million American children under the age of 17. I've heard parents say to me, "It seems like a lot more kids have asthma." You know what? They're right! The rate of asthma among children has increased by about 72 percent between 1982 and 1994. Most experts are attributing this to a dramatic increase in environmental toxins in our cities and towns.

Asthma can begin at any age, but most children experience their first attack before age four or five. In the early years, 10–15 percent of boys and 7–10 percent of girls develop asthma. By adolescence, the girls' rate catches up to the boys' until adulthood. Half of children are free from asthma by the time they are 20 years old, but can relapse into attacks with stress, poor diet, and a decline in overall health. The proper management and prevention for your child is essential in order to avoid a lifetime of breathing problems.

The cost of pediatric asthma is stunning, on a personal and on a national level. Take a look at these statistics:

➤ The cost in medical care and lost wages to families dealing with an asthmatic child exceeds $1.9 billion in this country alone.

➤ Forty-three percent of the asthma costs are from emergency room visits and hospitalization.

➤ American families who have children with asthma spend 5.5–14.5 percent of their income on asthma care.

➤ Ten million school days are missed each year due to asthma.

Trigger Checklist

Conventional scientists do not fully understand why your child becomes sensitive to certain substances and develops asthma. We do know 80 percent of children with asthma also have allergies. Pay close attention to your child's reaction around the following items and activities. Initially your child's reaction to a substance may be mild and may not even show up for as much as 20 hours after exposure. Continued exposure usually creates severe reactions over time.

Here are just a few of the many known allergy and asthma triggers:

➤ Dust mites   ➤ Pollen

➤ Pets   ➤ Cigarette smoke

➤ Cockroaches   ➤ Vegetable proteins

➤ Viruses

➤ Molds

➤ Exercise

➤ Cold air

➤ Castor bean protein

➤ Pollution

➤ Strong odors and perfumes

➤ Drugs like aspirin and ibuprofen

Oriental Medicine's Answer to Asthma

Your child's individual symptoms of asthma determine the oriental diagnosis and treatment plan used. One of the most common pediatric asthma conditions that I see in my office translates into deficient spleen asthma. Weak digestion and excessive mucus characterize this. The cough produces a lot of phlegm, poor appetite, bloated upper abdomen, pale complexion, fatigue, loose or incomplete stools, and pale tongue.

When faced with this diagnosis, your acu-pro will probably decide to perform acupuncture, usually stimulating points by gentle insertion without leaving the needles in place. The acupoints used will be very similar to the ones used in adults as seen in Chapter 12. Herbal formulas may be administered in eyedroppers. There are a vast assortment of formulas to fit your child's individual symptoms. Diet is especially important in this type of asthma. Too many cold, raw foods, or sugary foods can further injure your child's digestion, which will add to the accumulation of mucus that loads up the airways in asthma.

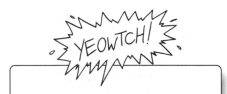

Harm Alarm

Don't smoke around your children! According to a 1999 study performed in Sweden, second-hand smoke may cause asthma. Children exposed to environmental tobacco smoke (ETS) in the home are twice as likely to be diagnosed with asthma. ETS was reported 21 percent more often than other asthma triggers.

Infant Massage for Asthma

Chinese Tui-Na (see Chapter 5, "Acupuncture—Tools of the Trade,") is used for infants as well as adults and can be quite helpful in relieving asthma. During the massage, rub gently into the acu-points CV-17, BL-12, and Ding Chuan which are discussed in Chapter 12, "Respiration—A Breath of Fresh Air," for asthma. Using a few drops of oil can reduce friction and make a more enjoyable time to connect with your baby. Soft singing is encouraged.

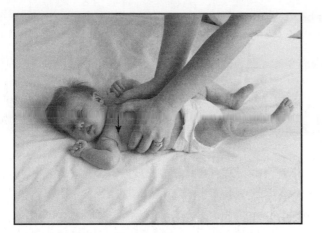

Massaging an asthmatic infant.

Rest your baby on a blanket while you place your hands, palm down, at the center of his or her chest. Gently push out to the sides, following the baby's little ribs. Review Chapter 12 for acu-points to softly press along the way. As your hands move to the sides, stay connected and move back up to the center of the chest. Repeat several times to increase circulation and release the tight chest muscles.

Diarrhea: Squirts for the Squirts

Most children will experience a short bout of diarrhea for one or two days occasionally, and such events are perfectly normal. However, persistent diarrhea that continues over a longer period of time can be a warning sign of your child's overall health. Take a look at Chapter 19 that focuses on gastrointestinal conditions for a discussion of the conventional medical causes and issues surrounding diarrhea.

In Oriental Medicine, the characteristics of the diarrhea and your child's health determine diagnosis and treatment. Dehydration is a concern with the loss of fluids. This results in oriental medicine as a deficient yin condition. You'll notice that your child has a dry mouth, dry skin, and red lips and tongue. The diarrhea will be yellowish, and the amount of urination will be less than you would expect.

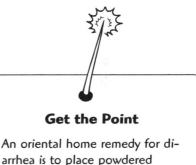

Get the Point

An oriental home remedy for diarrhea is to place powdered cloves and cinnamon bark in the child's navel and cover with an adhesive bandage. Keep in place for one to two hours, making sure the skin is not irritated. Repeat for a day or two. If this has not helped, call your health-care practitioner.

Acupuncture and herbs can be very effective in persistent diarrhea, because the symptoms, as well as the underlying Oriental Medical conditions, are treated. Dehydration can cause serious complications if left untreated. Seeking assistance can help your child's overall health improve. Acu-pros perform pediatric acupuncture using a gentle stimulation of acu-points mostly on the abdomen and legs. Each practitioner has his or her own techniques and will be sensitive to the fact that your baby is uncomfortable and will not hold still for prolonged procedures. Your baby will relax just as you would following a treatment and the relief will be shared by you both.

Nutritional Support: Awful Dophilus and More

Diet is incredibly important in treating persistent pediatric diarrhea. Food allergies such as wheat gluten, sugar malabsorption, or deficient pancreatic enzymes are the most common causes of this condition. Try cutting out wheat products for several weeks. (And check your labels; wheat is in everything!) Next, give sugary foods and juices some time off. Children often become addicted to sugar, so this may not be easy, but their improved health will strengthen your resolve.

I also recommend bland food selections of cooked or warmed foods. Eliminate cold and frozen foods or liquids and cut back on raw foods that can tax a struggling digestive system. Chinese herbs prescribed by a qualified herbalist can also be used successfully to stop the frequent flow. I also recommend a nutritional supplement called acidophilus, which replaces the healthy bacteria that are frequently lost in diarrhea. These good guys will aid absorption in your child's bowels and help stop persistent diarrhea. One of the children I treat whose front tooth was taken by the tooth fairy said she liked taking the "awful-dophilus" because it made her feel good!

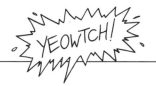

Harm Alarm

Watch your child with care if he or she suffers from diarrhea. Abdominal bloating, cramping, thin or watery stools, urgency, and occasional nausea characterize mild diarrhea. If you notice blood or mucus in the stools, sudden vomiting, weight loss, and fever, this suggests dysentery or infectious diarrhea. This is a more serious illness, and you should contact your healthcare provider immediately.

Add Just a Pinch: Pediatric Back Massage

Lay your child, tummy down, on a blanket or across your lap. Gently pinch and lift the loose skin over the spine. Work your way from the bottom to the top, loosely lifting the skin, talking, singing, and loving your child. This stimulates the acu-points along the spine, which leads to all the major organs. The pinch and lift is soft and gentle and will relax and soothe your child.

Ear Infections: The Fear Not to Hear

I've yet to meet a parent who doesn't dread the feverish, ear-tugging terrors that ear infections can bring to an otherwise happy baby. *Otitis media* (middle ear infection) is the most common form of ear infection. There were 30 million doctor visits for otitis media in 1997, which is up three-fold since 1975. Your conventional physician monitors your child's ears for any sign of fluid, redness, or inflammation, which could signal an increase in harmful bacteria. Antibiotics are usually the standard treatment in these situations.

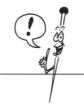

Acu-Moment

The American Academy of Pediatrics distinguishes between two kinds of **otitis media:**

➤ Acute otitis media. Symptoms include fever, ear pain, and pus behind the eardrum. Most doctors use antibiotics to treat this type.

➤ Otitis media with effusion. This condition involves fluid in the middle ear, which can cause temporary hearing loss that will return as the fluid drains. Antibiotics are not necessary to treat this. Your physician can monitor the ears to make sure the fluid is draining.

Unfortunately, the cycle of antibiotic use for recurrent ear infections can be maddening. As soon as the antibiotic treatment is finished, another ear infection pops up and it's off to the doctor's office for more meds. If the fluid does not drain, tubes are surgically implanted in your child's eardrum to prevent possible hearing loss.

Most ear infections occur in children between three months and three years old. The infections that I hear most often occur when a mother changes from breast milk to formula, starts feeding her baby solid foods, or when the baby starts teething. The fear is that improper hearing under the age of three may delay or impair normal language skills. It's a tricky time in most parents' lives. Oriental Medicine has a great deal to offer you to end the cycle of ear infections and help your baby's first years be healthy and happy ones.

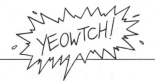

Harm Alarm

We'll say it again: Stop smoking! The August 1999 issue of *Pediatrics* reported on an Australian research study of ear infections from birth to age 5. This study compared children born to smoking and nonsmoking mothers.

➤ 1–9 cigarettes per day—60 percent higher risk for ear infections

➤ 10–19 cigarettes per day—260 percent higher risk for ear infections

➤ 20 or more cigarettes per day—330 percent increased risk for their child to develop ear infections

Ending the Cycle of Ear Infections: Stopping the Drama

Antibiotics can and do kill disease-causing bacteria. The physicians that I've worked with are doing their best to help your child. Studies show that otitis media resolves itself—without the need for any medication—within 14 days in about 80 percent of children. Using antibiotics increases the percentage to 95 percent. Antibiotics make the fluid in your child's ear sterile, but they do not make it go away. Oriental Medicine seeks to stimulate your child's immune system so that if you do use antibiotics, the next cold will not result in an ear infection. Individual characteristics are observed as in an adult and a comprehensive treatment plan is devised to end the infections and improve overall health.

I know how frustrating recurrent ear infections can be. Here are a few ways you can help to ease the ears:

➤ **Be a team player with your doctor.** Ask which kind of ear infection your child has and whether an antibiotic is necessary. Ask for periodic monitoring of your child's ears (the wait-and-watch method).

➤ **Get rid of the gluten.** Wheat snacks and breads often cause food allergies for our little ones.

➤ **Send out the sugar.** According to oriental medicine, sugar weakens the digestion. Cold ice cream and sweet fruit drinks add more impairment. By cutting back on sugar, you'll see the difference.

➤ **Leave the milk behind.** Many children do not tolerate cow's milk. Try fortified soy milk as a substitute; it doesn't contain the substances most likely to cause allergies, but still offers plenty of calcium.

➤ **Bring in the good guys.** Supplement your child's diet with the helpful, naturally occurring bacteria acidophilus and bifidus. They come in odorless, colorless, and tasteless powders that you can put in any liquid to boost immunity. Interestingly enough, bifidus is a key component of breast milk.

➤ **Send in the herbs.** Your acu-pro can work up a custom herbal formula for your baby to address the symptoms as well as the underlying weakness in his or her system.

I have seen these steps work quite well with recurrent ear infections. But they're not magic, and it takes time and patience to clear up the condition. As it stands now, your child's immune system has been weakened by frequent antibiotic use, often leaving him or her open to another infection or to developing antibiotic-resistant bacteria. The best results I've experienced come from coordinating your team of physician, acu-pro, and you. They are all working to help ensure your child gets the best care possible.

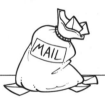

Mailbag

You'd think Katie was running for Town Mayor the way she smiled, greeted, and engaged everyone in the office during her first visit. The only obstacle barring this buoyant bouncing girl from office was that she was only 15 months old. Her parents had been dealing with chronic ear infections since they switched from breast milk to formula. She would start the typical tugging of her ear; her mood would become uncharacteristically sullen and withdrawn. At some point she began to cry and could not be consoled. This was their first child and they looked a little worn out, too. We began by going over Katie's medical history, including her mother's pregnancy. Sometimes unusual experiences or emotions strongly felt by the mother during pregnancy can be clues to a child's pattern of illness. We reviewed the formulas and snacks that they gave her, along with the juices and water she got throughout the day. I prescribed an herbal formula, which was administered in a dropper, and instructed both parents in how to give an ear massage to Katie. I suggested they do this nightly as part of a bedtime routine, and especially if she was pulling on her ears. We cut out quite a bit of dairy, wheat gluten, and sugars from her diet. Her parents were shocked by the amount she used to eat when we wrote it all down. Working with her pediatrician, Katie is now off the low-dose antibiotic she was scheduled to be on for almost a year and she's back impressing the crowds with her winning personality.

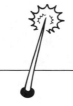

Get the Point

Compress for success. Use hot and cold compresses on the infected ear. Begin with a hot compress to improve circulation, adding the cold to reduce inflammation. Repeat several times a day for a few days in a row as needed, to bring comfort to your child.

Vomiting of Milk

There's a reason that parents of infants pack for a trip to the grocery store as if they were going on a year-long trek. You need to have a change of clothing for yourself and your child in case the vomiting doesn't hit your burp cloth smack in the middle, which it rarely does! This is especially true with breastfed babies who can become overwhelmed with the amount of milk when it finally "lets down" from the breast. If your child repeatedly vomits during or after a feeding, there may be a recognizable pattern brewing, and your acu-pro can save you some cleanup time and trouble.

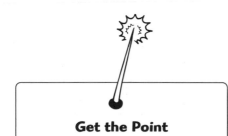

Get the Point

Make a tea from grating a few slices of fresh ginger and dried orange peel with hot water. Let steep five minutes, cool, and give one or two eyedroppers to your child before feeding. This will settle the stomach and help prevent further vomiting.

Determined Digestion: What Goes Down Can Stay Down

The most common form of vomiting is known in oriental terms as a deficient cold stomach. This is reflected in your baby's characteristics, such as vomiting back milk that he or she has just swallowed. It looks just like milk and usually has no change in color or odor. Your baby's hands and feet are usually cold, face is pale, and there often is a visible blue vein at the bridge of the nose. Your baby is usually less energetic than you might think and is uncomfortable if you put any pressure on his or her abdomen.

Chinese herbal medicines are designed to improve digestion and overall condition and health. I also recommend that mothers feed these children small, frequent amounts of milk rather than give them a few big feedings. If your child is eating solid foods, avoid cold or raw foods, which may overtax the digestive system. Toddlers quickly develop a taste for fatty, greasy foods like chips, fried foods, or peanut butter. Cutting out these items, despite the protests, will often resolve the vomiting and indigestion challenges.

All the pediatric conditions mentioned in this chapter weigh heavily on parents' minds as they do their best to care for the new life they've been blessed with. Oriental Medicine has been assisting parents for centuries in these common, but frustrating ailments. I will stress here again to work in concert with the other health care professionals that care for your child. Using the best and safest options is what everyone wants for your baby. Next we will look at the treatment options that are available to assist people with cancer.

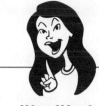

Wise Words

Projectile vomiting launches out of your child's mouth with great force, traveling amazing distances. Overfeeding and gulping of milk often are the cause, but if this continues, it could be a sign of gastroesophageol reflux disorder or pyloric stenosis. See your physician to rule these out.

The Least You Need to Know

➤ Crimping colic involves backing off gas-producing foods and overfeeding.

➤ Bond with your baby during a healing tummy massage for unwanted colic or constipation.

➤ Eighty percent of children with asthma also have allergies. Learn the list of asthma triggers to keep your child breathing better.

➤ Custom herbal prescriptions combine cinnamon, cloves, and other herbs to put a halt to persistent diarrhea.

➤ Coordinate Oriental Medicine with eliminating foods that might be causing allergic reactions, such as wheat, milk, and sugar.

➤ Feeding your baby smaller amounts of food or milk on a more frequent basis can significantly reduce vomiting during or after mealtime.

Chapter 15

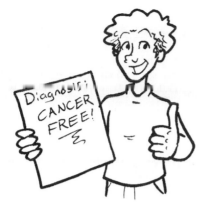

Cancer—A Ray of Hope

In This Chapter

➤ What is cancer?

➤ Discover how acu-points can stop chemotherapy-induced nausea and vomiting

➤ Acupressure to soothe tired and achy pain

➤ Let acu-points stimulate your immune system

➤ Learn how to keep your hair and increase your energy with Oriental Medicine

The treatment of cancer is one of the best examples of how conventional medicine and traditional Oriental Medicine can be integrated for the patient's well-being. Patients who consult with me for various types of cancer treatments have already been through the diagnostic process with their conventional physicians; some have begun treatment, while others are gathering information and options.

For some, it's their first journey into a vast array of therapies known as complementary medicine. They are often overwhelmed by the choices, promises, and practices of unfamiliar ways to heal their minds and bodies. The challenge I've encountered is finding a balance between conventional and complementary care, while limiting the number of therapies used at any one time, so valid evaluation is possible regarding the success of each specific treatment. A further challenge involves maintaining strong and open lines of communication between the patient and providers. I usually ask patients for permission to write a letter or make a phone call to their physicians. This opens up communication and fosters understanding for the overall benefit of the ones who have entrusted us with their care during one of the most challenging times in their lives.

This chapter will help you understand the hopeful options and choices that Oriental Medicine can bring to your treatments.

Cancer: The Conventional View

Our bodies are amazing in the way trillions of cells are made and distributed throughout a complex network of systems. Normal cells grow, reproduce, and die in response to internal and external signals from our body. When normal cells mutate or change into cancer cells, then the problem begins.

Cancer is the abnormal growth, reproduction, and spread of body cells. These cells do not obey the normal signals of the body that control other cells, and behave independently instead of working in harmony with your system. Sometimes cancer cells reproduce and form a lump or tumor. If the tumor is self-contained and doesn't spread, it's called benign and is usually surgically removed. If tumor cells grow, divide, damage the normal cells around them, and invade other tissue or travel through your bloodstream, the cells are called malignant or cancerous. Metastasis refers to a malignant tumor's cells that enter the bloodstream. The danger comes from the spread of these cancer cells to other tissues in your body, where new tumors can grow.

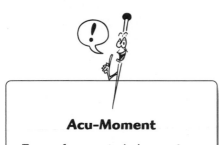

Acu-Moment

Types of cancer include **carcinomas,** which originate in the skin, lining of organs, and glands; **leukemias,** which are cancers of blood-forming tissues; **sarcomas,** which begin in connective tissue, bone, and cartilage; and **lymphomas,** which affect the lymphatic or immune system.

As tumors grow and multiply, they rob your normal healthy cells of nutrients, disrupting your body's ability to function. Deteriorating health or death usually results. No one knows exactly why some cells become cancer cells. Exposure to certain substances and particular lifestyle habits are linked to cancer development. For instance, we all know that exposure to cigarette smoke puts you at a significantly higher risk of lung cancer. A diet that is high in fat and low in fiber is associated with increased risk of colorectal cancer and is a factor in breast and prostate cancer, too.

There are more than 100 different diseases classified as cancers. In the United States, skin cancer is the most frequently diagnosed cancer, followed by breast, lung, prostate, colon and rectal, bladder, uterine, oral, leukemia, and pancreatic cancer, respectively.

Defining Your Cancer

Doctors diagnose cancer by using four factors that help define where the tumor is located and the progress it's made in your body:

➤ **Site.** The place where the cancer occurs (for example, lung, skin, breast).

➤ **Stage.** How much the tumor has grown or spread. There are four stages: Stage 1, contained to original site; Stage 2, spread to nearby lymph nodes or tissues; Stage 3, spread to other tissues in your body; Stage 4, spread to a large amount of tissue.

➤ **Grade and type.** The particular characteristics of your cancer (for example, aggressive and quick spreading, slow and not likely to spread to other tissues). These two factors are often linked because they share the same descriptive qualities.

Acupuncture: Improving Your Quality of Life

I focus on three main areas of concern when working with patients during their cancer treatment: nausea and vomiting from chemotherapy, cancer pain, and the stimulation of the immune system. I will also point out that I do not encourage patients to use Oriental Medicine to the exclusion of their oncologist or primary physician. I encourage clear communication between the patient's physicians and myself to ensure the best care.

While there are studies to support what most acupuncturists experience in their clinics, more research and integrated programs are needed. Expanding our knowledge will give practitioners and patients the confidence to use acupuncture in the most appropriate and effective ways.

Chemotherapy-Induced Nausea and Vomiting

Patients tell me how difficult it is to deal with all the emotions and logistics of chemotherapy, but the nausea and vomiting that often follow are just too much to bear. Your energy level and appetite decline rapidly. Antiemetic (antinausea) medications are available, but they may not work to alleviate the problem completely.

Studies show that acupuncture can be used effectively alone for nausea or provide added relief when using antiemetic treatments. I have found that acupuncture is highly effective in this area, and it's a real pleasure to bring relief to my patients during a difficult time in their lives. If you decide to add acupuncture to your treatment plan, expect your practitioner to use acu-points such as PC-6 (see the photo later in this chapter), ST-36 (see Chapter 16), and SP-4 (see Chapter 19). These acu-points all work well for calming down and rebalancing the digestive system.

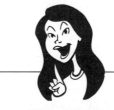

Wise Words

According to the National Institute of Health's panel of scientists, researchers, and practitioners, clinical studies on humans have shown acupuncture to be effective for nausea caused by cancer chemotherapy.

149

As a patient's condition improves, I normally give him biomagnets to use daily as part of his self-care program. Acupuncturists have been using magnets as part of their toolbox for years. Since studies have begun to suggest that an aspect of Qi energy can be manipulated with magnets, new and more convenient forms of magnet treatments have been available to your acu-pro. I have found that patients enjoy being active participants in their care and this easy, convenient, and effective treatment enables me to satisfy their wishes.

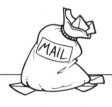

Mailbag

Beth was 44 years of age and undergoing chemotherapy treatments for breast cancer. Dealing with the cancer was hard enough, but the nausea and vomiting from the chemo were beginning to take their toll. She had tried antiemetic medications, but none had worked well for her. We began acupuncture treatments once a week and twice on the week she received chemo. She began to feel relief after the second visit and improved steadily afterward. When she did feel sick following her chemo, the symptoms were tolerable and did not last as long. We followed up with home acupressure and biomagnet therapy. Her appetite and energy returned, enabling her to be more comfortable during her course of cancer treatments.

Pain, Pain, Go Away

Acupuncture activates the opioid (painkilling) systems of our bodies. You will most likely feel relaxed and comfortable after your treatment, partly due to the release of these natural substances into your bloodstream. Research has been able to identify several opioids that flow into your central nervous system during acupuncture treatment and thereby reduce pain. Your individual treatment will depend on the location and type of cancer you have. Acupuncture is not done on or around the tumor site. The Qi channels that traverse your body are stimulated to safely relax muscles and decrease the pain that often accompanies cancer.

Boosting Your Immune System

Keeping yourself as healthy as possible during your treatments for cancer is vital to a successful outcome. Acupuncture can be used along with your treatments to maintain overall health. Our immune system is often measured by the percentage of T lymphocyte cells (particularly T-4) that are part of our body's natural resistance and immunity.

Studies are beginning to show a significant increase in T-4 cells following acupuncture therapy.

Your acu-pro will have also done a thorough initial visit to be able to assist you in general health and life quality. Many patients are finding that adding an acupuncturist to their cancer treatment team helps them feel better during the process of healing.

Healing Hands: Acupressure and Reflexology

The benefits of a healing touch can bring about much-needed relaxation, may reduce pain, encourage lymph flow, reduce edema, decrease nausea, and improve sleep. Acupressure and foot reflexology (see Chapter 3, "The Origins of Oriental Medicine") can help you feel more in control and assist you in adjusting to body changes from surgery, chemotherapy, and cancer. According to *Massage Magazine* (March/April 2000), patients who are touched during treatment experience a greater sense of relaxation and less insomnia, nausea, anxiety, depression, pain, and need for medication.

There are some considerations to keep in mind when giving self-acupressure or getting a treatment from a friend or practitioner:

➤ Avoid therapy on the specific site of the cancer. This can aggravate your pain.

➤ Do not use direct pressure on sites that contain a surgical wound, redness, or inflammation from radiation treatment. There may also be body positions that are uncomfortable while you are receiving a treatment.

➤ Be aware of the amount of pressure that you use. Use light to moderate pressure, especially if you are receiving chemotherapy treatments. Comfort is important to the overall effect, and chemotherapy places a heavy toxin load on the body. Be gentle.

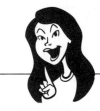

Wise Words

The National Cancer Institute of the National Institutes of Health endorses the use of massage, pressure, and vibration for musculoskeletal pain in cancer patients during all phases of treatment.

➤ Finally, let your physician know that you are receiving acupressure therapy and ask for any input regarding your sessions. Speaking with your physician affords a chance for both of you to learn.

Bodywork, which can be loosely defined as any kind of therapy that touches your skin, is being used throughout North America in private clinics, hospitals, and medical centers as part of a comprehensive treatment plan for cancer patients. Stanford University Hospital has been offering it since 1993. Shadyside Hospital Center for Complementary Medicine in Pittsburgh, Pennsylvania, offers shiatsu as well as

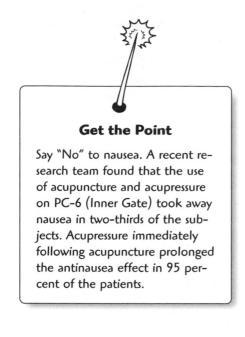

Get the Point

Say "No" to nausea. A recent research team found that the use of acupuncture and acupressure on PC-6 (Inner Gate) took away nausea in two-thirds of the subjects. Acupressure immediately following acupuncture prolonged the antinausea effect in 95 percent of the patients.

acupuncture and Chinese medicine as components of the center's protocol for cancer patients. Touching a cancer patient not only helps with the physical symptoms; touching also brings a sense of caring and acceptance that only the healing hands of another can bring.

Points used to treat pain may include any of the points that control the region of the pain. Remember that acu-points are selected for their effect on a region either locally, adjacent, or distal. For instance, with colon cancer you may not want to needle directly on the abdomen, but may treat the pain safely and effectively by using points on the arms and legs. This is the great advantage that working with acu-points and channels has over other therapies. Additional acu-points to help with nausea and boost the immune system are PC-6 (Inner Gate), ST-36, SP-6, and SP-4, which have been discussed earlier in this chapter.

Apply firm and steady pressure for one to three minutes to the acu-point that follows the median nerve and flexor tendons into the hand. Acu-point PC-6 (Inner Gate) is located three-fingers' width from the wrist crease.

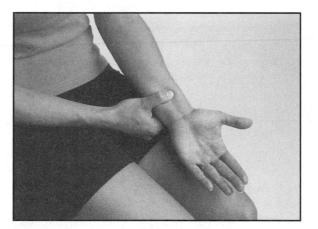

Chinese Herbal Medicine

The word "cancer" is never mentioned in the early Chinese medical texts. Cancer is a Latin derivative of the Greek word *karkinoma* or "crab," which describes the crab-like pattern of tumors. Chinese medicine does describe diagnostics and treatments for hard masses and tumors.

A qualified herbalist will conduct a thorough exam as outlined in Chapter 2, "What to Expect on Your First Visit—Does It Hurt?" and help you put together a comprehensive herbal and perhaps nutritional program. Chinese herbal medicine is extremely versatile and can be adapted to an individual's specific cancer and his or her reaction to the process. Herbal prescriptions can be updated and modified as your condition changes, so you will always be receiving herbs to match your needs.

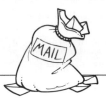

Mailbag

Francine was 42 years of age and had just been diagnosed with breast cancer. She had chosen to combine conventional and complementary medicines. I used acupuncture during her initial chemotherapy, which eliminated any nausea she felt from the cancer treatments. I wrote a customized herbal prescription to help her with general energy and digestion complications, as well as retention of her hair. While her friends in the hospital support group became weak and lost their hair, Francine remained vital and experienced no hair loss, only thinning. She continued with acupuncture and herbs throughout her cancer treatment and was able to work and interact with her family. This was her goal. I have just seen her two years later, and she's still going strong!

I've had patients say to me many times that they would never choose to have to deal with cancer; however, the life-changing experience has brought them closer to what is truly important in their lives. They hope that richness will inspire them to share a full and loving experience with their family and friends. I have been thankful that Oriental Medicine has been able to help improve the quality of life for so many. From here we move to the beginnings of life in the next chapter, "Birthing Baby." I'll describe the helpful therapies available to you and yours from getting pregnant and morning sickness to bouncing back from giving birth.

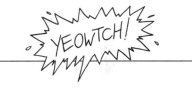

Harm Alarm

Avoid those chemicals! Many chemicals promote free radicals in your body, which only lead to cancer. Limit your use of any products from an aerosol can and avoid hairsprays, cleaning compounds, pesticides, and paints.

The Least You Need to Know

➤ Cancer is the abnormal growth, reproduction, and spread of body cells.

➤ There are more than 100 different diseases that are classified as cancer.

➤ Acupuncture can significantly reduce cancer pain and boost immunity.

➤ Recent research showed chemotherapy-induced nausea and vomiting was reduced in 95 percent of patients who used acupuncture and acupressure.

➤ Acupressure and reflexology increase relaxation and the ability to sleep, and may reduce edema, anxiety, disease, and nausea.

➤ Chinese herbal medicine is extremely versatile and can be customized to fit your individual cancer treatments.

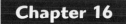

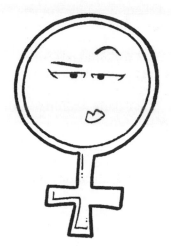

Chapter 16

Birthing Baby

In This Chapter

➤ Finding viable solutions for female infertility

➤ Use acu-points to end morning sickness

➤ Childbirth made easier ... even breech

➤ After giving birth, discover how Oriental Medicine helps you get back on your feet

---

"I'm pregnant!" "I'm in the family way!" "I've got a bun in the oven!" These are just a few of the ways you may share the happy news that the miracle of life is happening inside you.

This chapter is for all women who either want to say those happy words or are facing the nauseating challenges of morning sickness. For those who are planning their childbirth experience, take a closer look at the many benefits that your acu-pro can bring to you for inducing a comfortable labor. If you've recently been there and done that, make sure to explore how Oriental Medicine rebuilds your body after childbirth. Keep on reading: There's a little something for everyone who aspires to motherhood.

Female Infertility: The Obstruction to Reproduction

For most couples, getting pregnant isn't a problem, but one in five couples experience fertility issues in America today. The risk for infertility among women 35–44 years of age is double that of women 30–34 years of age, and the risk is one-and-a-half times

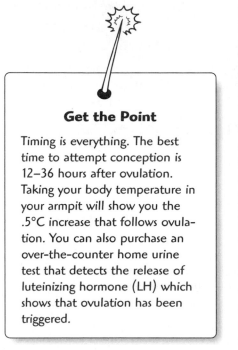

Get the Point

Timing is everything. The best time to attempt conception is 12–36 hours after ovulation. Taking your body temperature in your armpit will show you the .5°C increase that follows ovulation. You can also purchase an over-the-counter home urine test that detects the release of luteinizing hormone (LH) which shows that ovulation has been triggered.

higher for black women than for white women. Doctors usually define infertility as the inability to conceive after a year or more of regular sexual activity without contraception during the time of ovulation. It also encompasses an inability to carry a pregnancy to full term. Needless to say, infertility is an emotionally painful, financially draining, and physically exhausting condition.

Getting pregnant isn't as easy as it looks. Indeed, there are a host of intricate processes that must be completed during ovulation, fertilization, and implantation of eggs into the uterus. Most of the couples I see have already been through a battery of tests to determine the possible causes of infertility. These conditions range from failure to ovulate properly to polycystic ovaries, blocked fallopian tubes, endometriosis, uterine fibroids, sexually transmitted disease, and pituitary, thyroid, or adrenal disorders. Emotions such as fear, anxiety, anger, and resentment are often by-products of this stressful time in a couple's inability to conceive.

This chapter discusses female infertility; however, it is equally important for men to be examined for low sperm count, motility, or anatomical abnormalities that may contribute to inability to conceive.

Improving the Odds with Oriental Medicine

I prefer to meet with both partners to discuss their fertility options with Oriental Medicine. We discuss the diagnosis they received from their conventional physician, the course of therapy or medication they have tried, and their current stress levels, which can run quite high under these circumstances. I'll then proceed with the oriental diagnostic process outlined in Chapter 2, "What to Expect on Your First Visit—Does It Hurt?" to determine the patterns of imbalance that, in traditional medicine, lead to problems with conception.

One of the most common conditions is infertility due to cold in the uterus. This condition is characterized by delayed menstruation with dark flow, pain, and coldness in the lower abdomen and limbs, sore back, weak knees, and profuse, clear urine. Warming herbs and moxibustion may be used with acupuncture to treat this condition. These are all symptoms of cold that would hamper the flow of Qi, which is essential for normal function to occur in organs. These techniques are designed to restore normal function and flow of energy while creating the best possible environment in which a new life can thrive.

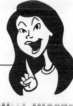

Wise Words

Research published in a 1994 issue of *The American Journal of Epidemiology* suggests that some women do not break down and absorb the sugar in milk (galactose). The presence of galactose in some women's blood can be harmful to unfertilized eggs. Have your blood tested to see if you are susceptible to this condition or, just to be on the safe side, curtail your intake of milk for several months and see what happens.

If your acu-pro works like I do, he or she will first make a diagnosis and assess the situation, then discuss the options available and outline a treatment plan. The goal, of course, is to create the best possible environment inside your body for a baby to grow, but of course there are no guarantees.

The good news is that, unlike many Western treatments for infertility that can be quite debilitating, you'll experience no side effects and will likely improve your overall health. Patience and clear communication with your acu-pro and conventional physician are essential for developing a safe and successful conception.

Acu-Points to Clear the Way

Your acu-pro will instruct you as to the exact points to press according to your individual diagnosis. Here are some of the most common acu-points that will fit into any acupressure session for infertility issues.

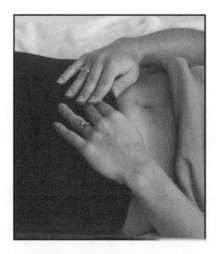

Fighting infertility.

Locate CV-6 (Sea of Qi) two-finger width directly below your navel, and CV-4 (Hinge at the Source), which is four-finger width directly below your navel. Press these points with firm pressure as you breathe deeply, concentrating on Qi filling your lower abdomen.

Additional acu-points used to treat infertility are discussed in Chapter 9, "Pain Below the Belt," and Chapter 17, "The Disappointment Down Under."

Morning Sickness: Easy to Be Queasy

So you're enjoying being pregnant, telling friends and family about the baby's new room, when suddenly your appetite plummets. This is followed by persistent nausea and vomiting. It's called morning sickness, but my patients tell me they can feel lousy any time of the day. About one-half of all pregnant women experience morning sickness at some point between weeks six and twelve. One out of 200 women will experience continuous nausea and vomiting that can result in dehydration, malnutrition, and unwanted weight loss.

Acu-Points to Bring Back Your Appetite

Being able to treat morning sickness makes me glad I'm an acupuncturist. Weak, tired, and frustrated expectant mothers come into the clinic, and generally within the first two treatments, they've noticed a big change. There are certainly herbs to use for nausea, but I have found that acupuncture works fast at thoroughly alleviating the symptoms so that you can get back to normal eating habits and enjoy your pregnancy.

Please note that there are some acu-points to avoid during pregnancy because they create circulation in the lower abdomen and uterus. A qualified acupuncturist learns these points in the first year of training and will safely and efficiently guide you through this challenging time of your pregnancy.

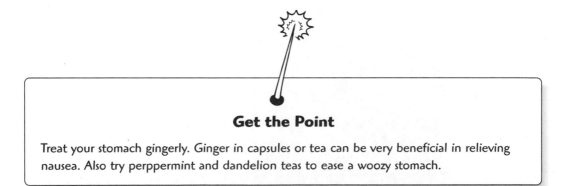

Get the Point

Treat your stomach gingerly. Ginger in capsules or tea can be very beneficial in relieving nausea. Also try perppermint and dandelion teas to ease a woozy stomach.

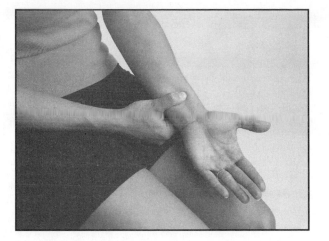

Easing morning sickness.

Apply firm and steady pressure for one to three minutes to the acu-points that follow the median nerve and flexor tendons into the hand. These acu-points include P-6 (Inner Gate), located two-finger widths from the wrist; P-7 (Big Tomb), located mid-point of the crease that runs across the wrist; and P-8 (Labor's Palace), located in the middle of the palm between the second and third bones of the hand.

Easing morning sickness.

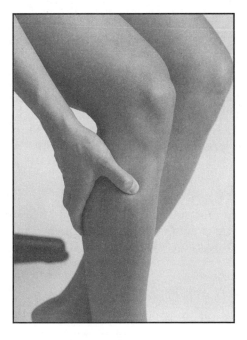

Locate ST-36 (Three Measures on the Leg), which is located about four-finger width below the kneecap and one-finger width to the outside. Use reinforced index and middle fingers, firmly pressing for one to two minutes. Breathe deep, gentle breaths, and rub the point after pressing.

159

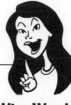

Wise Words

A malpositioned baby—also known as a breech baby—is the most common cause of difficult labor. Treatment by moxibustion (see Chapter 5, "Acupuncture—Tools of the Trade") has a long history of success at rotating the baby. This is done by simply heating the acupoint BL-67 (End of Yin) located on the outside of the nail on the little toe. One to five treatments usually does it. Stop the treatments after the baby has turned.

Childbirth: The Joy of Giving

Your due date is fast approaching. You've got your doctor, midwife, and place of delivery picked out, but what about your acu-pro? A growing number of women are choosing acupuncture to use throughout their pregnancy and as an optional treatment for an overdue or difficult labor.

Has your due date come and gone? Do you love being pregnant but had a difficult, prolonged labor with your last child? Who are you gonna call? Qi Busters! In all seriousness, this is a great choice for many mothers.

Marie was a patient of mine that I successfully treated during pregnancy for debilitating migraines. She did not do well with medications and was worried about using them to induce labor. When she saw her due date pass by, she came in for acupuncture therapy. I used needle and electro-acupuncture. Her cervix dilated following her first treatment, and after the second treatment, she delivered a healthy baby boy.

Acu-Points to Help You Pop

While you hurry up and wait during labor, use acu-points LI-4 and SP-6 to move things along. You'll need some help from your birthing team for the SP-6 point above your ankle—it'll probably be tough to reach.

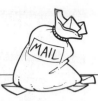

Mailbag

Jeff and Kathy were excited to be having their first baby. All the grandparents were fussing over Kathy, and Jeff was getting his share of slaps on the back by other fathers he knew. They were both attending birthing classes in preparation for the big day. They came to see me a little sad and disappointed following their last medical exam, during which they were informed their baby boy was in the breech position. He was healthy in all ways, but upside down in the womb. They stopped the birthing classes and Kathy resigned herself to an operation. They asked if anything could be done. I said that a moxa technique was commonly used to turn breech-positioned babies. They came to my office with Jeff's parents and I taught them all to do a simple, direct moxa burning therapy on Kathy's small toe. I explained to use this technique one to two times a day for five days, which coincided with a regularly scheduled apointment with their Ob-Gyn. I checked in with them to make sure they understood the instructions. They called me at the end of the week, relating the surprised look on their physician's face when he found that their baby had somehow flipped over and was in the perfect position for birth. They were able to have a normal birth experience, and as of the writing of this text, parents and baby were all doing fine.

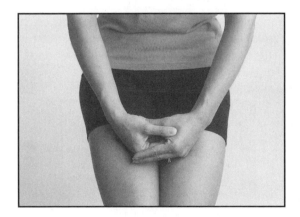

Moving things along in the delivery room.

Locate LI-4 (Adjoining Valleys) in the middle of the web between the thumb and index finger. This acu-point will be sore, but you'll need to press firmly anyway to jump-start delivery. Press for one to two minutes repeatedly until labor is underway.

*Moving things along in
the delivery room.*

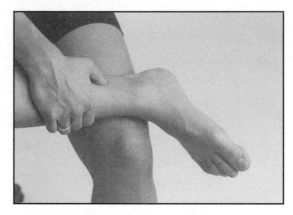

Locate SP-6 (Three Yin Junction) by measuring four-finger width above the tip of the inside ankle in the center of the leg. Press firmly for one to two minutes while the expectant mother continues to breathe deeply. Repeat several times until the blessed event occurs.

Bounce Back from Giving Birth

Your baby is healthy and beautiful. All your relatives want pictures e-mailed to them until they can come and visit. The doctors have fussed over your newborn, reassuring you that all is well. So what about you? You've just gone through an extremely rigorous nine-month workout that culminated in a whirlwind of emotions, physical strain, and tremendous blood loss. How are you going to bounce back so that you can resume life and care for an infant who needs you night and day?

Oriental Medicine has many helping hands to lend a new mother. Chinese herbs and food therapy are used to nourish and balance your body and improve your overall energy. Acupuncture helps heal the trauma your body goes through while restoring the normal function and flow of Qi in the channels.

*Getting back to normal
after childbirth.*

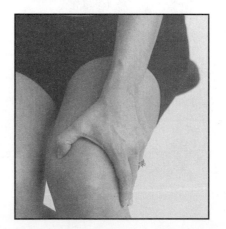

Locate SP-10 (Sea of Blood) by flexing your knee and measuring two-finger width above the inside of your kneecap. This point may be tender after childbirth, so press gently but firmly for one to two minutes. Repeat several times. Do this daily to restore normal menstruation and help lower abdominal bloating.

Part with Postpartum Depression

Postpartum depression affects approximately 10–20 percent of new mothers, and usually appears between two to eight weeks after delivery. This is different from postpartum blues (sadness, anxiety, insomnia, and weepiness) that appear within several days of delivery and go away in 10–12 days. The blues are common, affecting between 50 and 80 percent of all new mothers.

Postpartum depression can last from weeks to a year, and the symptoms may be intense and frightening to the new mother and her family. The risk factors for postpartum depression include a history of moderate to severe premenstrual syndrome and depression, among others.

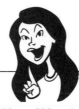

Wise Words

Risk factors for women with postpartum depression include

➤ History of moderate-to-severe PMS (premenstrual syndrome).

➤ Depression or anxiety during pregnancy.

➤ Family history of depression, anxiety, or substance abuse.

➤ Recent stressful event (family death, moving, job loss).

➤ Lack of emotional support.

➤ Low self-esteem.

➤ Long, complicated pregnancy.

➤ Newborn with physical or behavioral problems.

Oriental Medicine explains this condition as a sudden loss of blood and yin, which leaves the body unable to nourish and balance the mind and spirit. Your acu-pro will use acupuncture and acupressure, Chinese herbal medicines, and Qi Gong meditations to help you take back your life and feel good again. As usual, your exact condition will determine the treatment, but many of the herbs that you are likely to find in your prescription include Dang Gui, Shu Di Huang, Bai Shao, and Ye Jiao Teng. These can be prepared in teas, capsules, or powders, just to name a few. Acupuncture, acupressure, and Qi Gong are all designed to free up the heavy stagnant Qi that often accompanies this condition. Acupuncture is on the World Health Organization's list of viable treatments for depression.

The topics we've just discussed can be extremely emotional if you're in the middle of important decisions about the life and welfare of your family and yourself. I suggest taking a moment and weighing the options available to you. Oriental Medicine can be a valuable addition to your health team. We continue dealing with some of the most common and disruptive conditions that some women face. Stay with me, there's empowerment and assistance around the bend.

The Least You Need to Know

➤ Acu-pros can give renewed hope for couples struggling with fertility issues.

➤ Stop morning sickness with acupuncture or acupressure on P-6 (Inner Gate).

➤ Use acupuncture to avoid difficult or delayed labor.

➤ Breech babies can turn around following moxibustion on BL-67 (End of Yin).

➤ Get your strength and stamina back after childbirth with the help of Oriental Medicine.

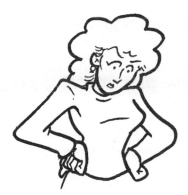

Chapter 17

The Disappointment Down Under

In This Chapter

➤ PMS gets put away

➤ Gain freedom from painful periods

➤ Successfully manage menopause

Jokes about premenstrual or menopausal women gone out of control are prevalent in our society. But to the women I see who are seeking help for these conditions, this is no laughing matter.

The not-so-funny part is that most women don't know that help is available for PMS, painful periods, and menopausal symptoms through Oriental Medicine. Real solutions exist that can improve the quality of your health, no matter what time of your life or the month it happens to be.

PMS (Premenstrual Syndrome)

One to two weeks before menstruation begins, your PMS symptoms make themselves known to you. Approximately 70–75 percent of women say they experience one or more of the following PMS symptoms some time in their lives: weight gain, breast tenderness, abdominal bloating, backache, joint pain, acne, cramps, fatigue, insomnia, anxiety, food cravings, and personality changes. Disruption of daily activities is reported by 30–40 percent of women, while 5 percent of women become completely disabled by PMS. Perimenopausal women may experience these symptoms well before and after the menstrual cycle.

Foods to Get You Back in the Saddle: The PMS Diet

One way to prevent, or at least alleviate, your premenstrual symptoms is to alter your daily diet, especially in the two weeks before your period starts. Some suggestions include the following:

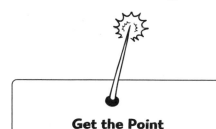

➤ Cut back on refined sugar, salt, red meat, junk foods, alcohol, coffee, tea, colas, and chocolate.

➤ Limit tobacco use.

➤ Eat more fish, poultry, whole grains, legumes (beans, peas, lentils), and high-protein snacks between meals.

➤ Reduce or eliminate dairy products.

➤ Increase consumption of green, leafy vegetables.

➤ Supplement with oils such as black currant seed, flaxseed, and evening primrose.

Get the Point

Keep your hormones on the level. Many women with PMS have elevated estrogen levels and low progesterone levels in the luteal phase of their menstrual cycle that follows ovulation. Adding B vitamins can help your liver inactivate estrogens. B_6 has been shown to elevate progesterone. Increasing dietary fiber and decreasing animal fats will also help free you from PMS.

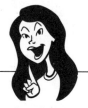

Wise Words

Studies suggest that women who regularly consume caffeine (coffee, tea, sodas, and chocolate) are four times more likely to develop severe PMS.

Ready, Aim, Press These Points for PMS

With a condition that has so many possible symptoms associated with it, women often experience the most relief after I find corresponding patterns that link these symptoms. This ability to find the connections between different bodily functions and malfunctions is certainly one of the strengths of Oriental Medicine. Your premenstrual headache, abdominal bloating, pain before your period, irritability, dark sides of your tongue, and a strong wiry quality to your pulse are all part of the stagnant Liver Qi diagnosis that your acupro will identify on your first visit. These symptoms may all be looked at as unrelated conditions in conventional medicine, but they fit an established pattern in Oriental Medicine, which has multiple treatment options ready to work for you.

A treatment plan including acupuncture can greatly relieve—if not completely eliminate—PMS from your life each month. I look forward to women telling me they no longer plan events around disabling PMS, and the whole month is theirs to use as they wish!

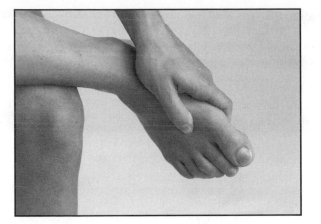

Easing PMS.

Locate LIV-3 (Great Pouring), which is above the webbing between the big toe and the second toe. Using the thumb, press firmly into the sorest spot for one or two minutes. Breathe deeply, repeating two to four times per session, one to two sessions a day.

Painful Periods: Dissing Dysmenorrhea

Primary dysmenorrhea, or painful menstrual periods, results from uterine muscle contractions as tissue passes through a narrow opening in the cervix. Secondary dysmenorrhea is associated with conditions such as endometriosis that may produce lesions that affect the reproductive cycle (see Chapter 18, "Female Frustrations"). Pain can be experienced before, during, or after menstruation.

Conventional medicine lists a tipped uterus, lack of exercise, and anxiety as contributing factors in dysmenorrhea. Oriental Medicine adds overwork, stress, chronic illness, excessive sexual activity, and improper recovery from childbirth as additional situations that contribute to monthly discomfort. Conventional medical treatments include applying local heat to the abdomen, drug therapy for pain, and in the case of secondary dysmenorrhea, correction of underlying abnormalities through surgery.

Oriental Medicine Helps the Flow Go

For dysmenorrhea, as for all conditions, your unique individual characteristics and overall health determine the appropriate Oriental Medical diagnosis and treatment plan. I tend to see a great deal of

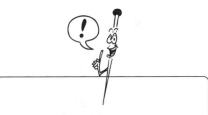

Acu-Moment

Menstrual is derived from the Latin word *menstrualis,* meaning "month." **Menses** is based on the Latin word *mensis,* derived from the Greek word for "month." These words were later used to describe the monthly flow of blood from the uterus.

167

women with conditions traditionally referred to as stagnation of cold in the lower abdomen. Their symptoms usually include pain that is present before or after the period in the center of the lower abdomen. The pain gets better with heat and gets worse from cold. Women with this type of condition tend to feel cold all over, have a sore lower back, and produce very little menstrual blood with dark clots.

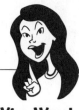

Wise Words

A research article published in the January 1987 issue of *Obstetrics and Gynecology* revealed that acupuncture can help alleviate primary dysmenorrhea. Ninety percent of the women who underwent regular acupuncture treatments designed to treat their painful periods showed improvement during this one-year study, while also being able to reduce their pain medications by 41 percent.

This condition responds well to acupuncture or acupressure, moxibustion, warming Chinese herbs, and the dietary guidelines listed earlier in this chapter. I encourage you to seek a qualified acu-pro for assistance with this common but treatable condition.

Relieving dysmenorrhea.

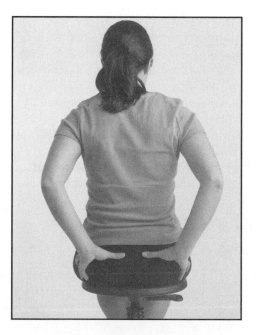

Locate BL-23 (Kidney Hollow) on the back following the middle of your waist until you're two-finger width to either side of your spine. Also find BL-31 and BL-34 (Eight Seams) pictured in the previous figure, which are located just below the bottom of the back, in the four holes in the sacrum. These acu-points affect painful menses and can be self-treated as shown in Chapter 9, "Pain Below the Belt." You can also place a hot water bottle on these spots for stagnation of cold, or have someone apply steady pressure for one to two minutes with heat. Repeat as needed for comfort.

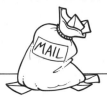

Mailbag

Mary doesn't schedule anything important during "that time of the month," she told me. Since she was a teenager, the two weeks after ovulation and before the beginning of her menses have held nothing but pain and discomfort. Her nerves are on end, breasts become sore and painful so sex with her husband is not enjoyable. The closer to the start of her period, the more intense the bloating, headaches, and irritability become. She had tried many medications, including birth control pills, but had always developed unwanted side effects after prolonged use. We began by using acupuncture once a week, with her doing home bio-magnetic treatments daily. She cut out a lot of the "comfort foods" like chocolate and dairy products, then added more protein from fish, veggies of the dark green leafy variety like spinach, and included flaxseed supplements once a day. She felt significant relief by the second cycle, and we added more acupressure techniques to her growing home routines. Her improvement was consistent over the next six months. I now see her only occasionally for other complaints and she is bringing her daughter for treatment so she can have help right away.

Menopause: The Hormonal Hostage

I've often heard women say that the change of life is one of the touchiest times in their lives. The body and mind that they have become accustomed to for 40+ years are now different and often unpredictable. This change is a natural transition in a woman's life as fertility comes to an end. Menopause refers to a point when a woman stops ovulating and menstruating. Pre- or perimenopause lasts about five to ten years before the last period. This transition is marked by irregular menstruation, showing the decline in your body's ovary production of the reproductive hormones estrogen and progesterone. Typically, the last period occurs around age 50. Hormone replacement therapy, or *HRT,* is the only satisfactory therapy that conventional medicine offers to relieve such symptoms as hot flashes. When estrogens are contraindicated because of a family history of breast cancer, other medications are prescribed to control symptoms.

169

Acu-Moment

HRT stands for hormone replacement therapy, which attempts to restore estrogen and progesterone to their premenopause levels. Using HRT is a personal choice and should be made after careful consideration of potential side effects or at-risk history for heart disease, breast or uterine cancers, or fibroid tumors. Read and ask your health provider questions before making one of the most important decisions at this stage of your life.

Menopausal symptoms vary with each individual woman. Some women barely notice the change while others feel drastic changes in normal daily life. Estrogen has effects on cells of the skin, breast, vagina, bladder, heart, liver, arteries, and brain.

The variety of symptoms women experience include hot flashes, night sweats, decreased sex drive, bladder problems, anxiety, depression, vaginal dryness and itching, breast tenderness, dry skin, fatigue, mood swings, poor memory, heart palpitations, and insomnia. For those that experience these bodily changes, it can be a real challenge.

YEOWTCH!

Harm Alarm

Stop smoking! Premature menopause is the early shutdown of the ovaries before age 40. Smoking is associated with this premature reduction in the estrogen level. Because estrogen is important in bone formation, smoking also puts you at risk for osteoporosis and health-jeopardizing bone fractures.

Press Acu-Points to Pause Your Menopause

The natural process of menopause has been getting comforting help from Oriental Medicine for centuries. As you've already read, diet, exercise, and a healthy outlook are key components of any comprehensive treatment plan. Hot flashes, dry skin, vaginal dryness, increased thirst, insomnia, forgetfulness, and anxiety are part of the deficient heart yin pattern in Oriental Medicine. The term "deficient yin" in this case often refers to the reduction in estrogen. The term "heart" addresses not only the organ itself, but the accompanying forgetfulness, insomnia, palpitations, and mood changes.

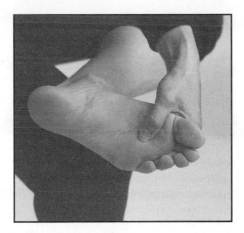

Pausing menopause.

Locate KD-1 (Gushing Spring) on the middle of the sole of your foot, one-third the distance from the base of your toes to the heel in a little hollow between muscles. While breathing deeply, apply firm pressure with your thumbs for one to two minutes. This acu-point helps clear your head and bring down your body temperature. This is a great point to press throughout the day to regain balance.

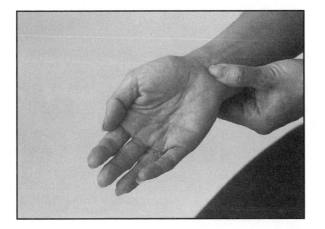

Pausing menopause.

Locate HT-7 (Spirit's Door) at the end of the wrist crease, up from the little finger on the palm side of the hand. Hold this point with your index finger, closing your eyes and breathing deeply to calm your mind and release tension.

Many of the conditions we've discussed here have been given more reasonable solutions partly due to better education and the growing demand for results. I'm glad that Oriental Medicine offers such possibilities for normal conditions that were just not talked about. We will continue our investigation into ways that acupuncture and acupressure can alleviate other gynecological problems.

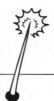

Get the Point

Stock up on soy! The British medical journal *Lancet* reported that Japanese women have fewer menopausal symptoms than American women, perhaps because they typically eat more plants containing substances called phytoestrogens. These substances are similar to the human estrogen women naturally produce. Today more than 2,000 soy products are on the market, including shakes, bars, and even coffee! Other sources of phytoestrogens are tofu, miso, flaxseed, and dates.

The Least You Need to Know

➤ Thirty to forty percent of women experience disruptive PMS.

➤ Cutting back on caffeine sources like coffee, tea, soda, and chocolate help curb PMS symptoms.

➤ Acu-points offer effective relief for painful periods.

➤ Menopause is a natural transition in life, not a disease.

➤ Calm nerves and release menopausal tension with acupressure on KD-1 and HT-7.

Part 4
Silent Sufferers

You're not wearing bandages, a plaster cast, or a sling, so you must not be hurt too bad. Without a reminder, your friends and family might forget you're dealing with a real health challenge. Sometimes other people don't understand that pain can be covered up as you try to live a normal life. Your pain doesn't always show. Most of the patients I've seen with the following conditions such as endometriosis, ovarian cysts, and chronic bladder infections have either a hard time finding the words for what is going on, or have given up reminding those around them. They often suffer in silence.

Well, I'm going to speak up about these conditions and the treatments that Oriental Medicine has waiting for you. Whether you're dealing with cysts, eczema, endometriosis, irritable bowel syndrome (IBS), or anxiety, get the help you need from these time-tested treatments. I know it's not always been easy. I encourage you to continue through the upcoming pages to discover a way to smile ... for real.

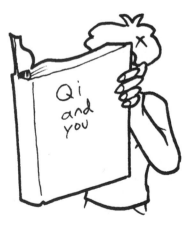

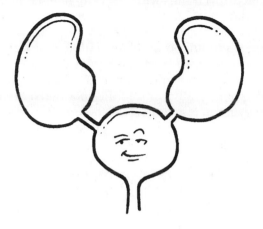
Female Frustrations

Have you ever felt like you were between a rock and a hard place? That's how endometriosis and uterine fibroids are frequently described to me by women who are at their wits' end for solutions to these hard problems. In Oriental Medicine, these conditions are most often described as hard masses, stagnant Qi, stuck blood, or phlegm. The strategies I use are designed to "soften" the hardness, and dissolve (if possible) or shrink the cysts and fibroids. Endometriosis symptoms can often be greatly reduced, and there is definite relief so your bladder doesn't bother you all the time. I look forward to sharing the possibilities that could change the quality of your life. Now it's time to begin the journey.

Endometriosis: Oh, the Tangled Webs We Weave

Endometriosis involves the growth of cells from the endometrium (the uterus lining) in other areas of your abdomen. About 12 million American women report having this condition—that's 10–20 percent of the female population.

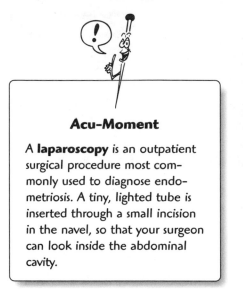

Acu-Moment

A **laparoscopy** is an outpatient surgical procedure most commonly used to diagnose endometriosis. A tiny, lighted tube is inserted through a small incision in the navel, so that your surgeon can look inside the abdominal cavity.

Endometriosis begins with a backup of endometrial tissue that builds up throughout the month during a regular menstrual cycle. The cause of this tissue backup is still unknown. Instead of flowing out of the uterus, some of the tissue moves back up through the fallopian tubes (which transport ovulated eggs) and falls out into the abdominal cavity. These living cells are often called implants, and they continue to respond to cyclical hormonal changes. They grow, build up, and bleed, just like they did before in the uterus, except there's nowhere for the blood to go. The blood can be absorbed slowly by the lining of the abdomen, but the remaining build-up of weblike tissue and blood clots causes the scarring and adhesions that can affect your fallopian tubes, ovaries, bladder, or bowel. A conventional Western doctor usually diagnoses endometriosis with *laparoscopy,* an outpatient surgical procedure that allows the doctor to examine your internal abdominal structures.

Endo Risks and Symptoms: Could This Be You?

While the causes of endometriosis are still unclear, here is a valuable list of the current medical thoughts on the condition:

➤ Deficiency in the immune system

➤ Family history of endometriosis

➤ Menstrual cycle length of 27 days or less

➤ Early onset of menstruation

➤ Periods lasting seven or more days

➤ Reported mostly by women who have never been pregnant

The symptoms of endometriosis can be difficult to evaluate. In the beginning, many women do not have *any* symptoms. Others who have severe buildup of tissue have no pain, while some women with only small adhesions have disabling discomfort. Although endometriosis is usually diagnosed between the ages of 25 and 35, the condition could begin about the same time that menstruation starts. Many of these symptoms are frequently ignored or thought of as a normal part of the cycle. Have a conversation with your healthcare provider if you experience any of these symptoms:

➤ Increasingly painful periods

➤ Severe pelvic cramps or abdominal pain one to two weeks before the menstrual period

➤ More frequent or irregular menses

➤ Pelvic or low-back pain felt at any time during the cycle

➤ Pain during or following sexual intercourse

➤ Pain with bowel movements

➤ Infertility (approximately 25–50 percent of these cases are due to endometriosis)

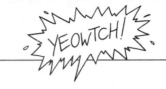

Harm Alarm

If you have symptoms of endometriosis, make sure you use a pad and not a tampon during menstruation. Tampons can increase pain and cramping during your cycle and may make reflux menstruation (the tissue backup) more likely.

Edging Out Endo: Acu-Points Plus

Endometriosis can be a stubborn and frustrating condition because of the complex interplay of hormones and unknown scarring and adhesions. Dr. Joel Hargrove, of Vanderbilt, Tennessee, has spent many years studying the effects of endometriosis. He states that PMS is reported by 80–90 percent of women with endometriosis. Conventional medical treatment is controversial and must be individualized. Medications are often prescribed to suppress ovarian function. Oral contraceptives may also be used in an attempt to prevent the proliferation of endometriosis. Side effects of suppressive medications, such as danazol, are often unpleasant and include weight gain, fluid retention, fatigue, decreased breast size, acne, hot flashes, and muscle cramps.

In my experience, Oriental Medicine can significantly improve a woman's menstrual cycle (see Chapter 17, "The Disappointment Down Under"). If adhesions are too numerous, surgery may be recommended, but reoccurrence of endometriosis is very high. So even if you have the tissue removed by laser surgery, it may very well grow back. I have found that acupuncture and herbal medicine have brought satisfactory relief to many of my patients for whom surgery is not indicated, not wanted, or has already been done.

In addition to treatment, I advise women to follow the PMS diet discussed in Chapter 17 and to exercise regularly. According to a report in *The Journal of the American Medical Association,* strenuous exercise lowers the levels of estrogen in the body, which may help the symptoms of endometriosis.

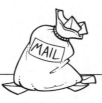

Mailbag

When I first met Anne, she was 37 years of age and had already undergone laser surgery for infertility due to endometriosis. She had still not been able to conceive, had adopted two little girls, and found her old endo symptoms returning. With two small children to care for, her downtime from abdominal pain, constipation, and nausea was more than she could bear. We began with acupuncture and herbs, such as Dang Gui, Mu Dan Pi, and Chi Shao that significantly reduced her symptoms after one month of treatment. After three cycles, she felt greatly improved, acupuncture treatments were reduced to the times just before and after ovulation, and she uses herbs, biomagnets, acupressure, and nutrition to stay feeling good. It takes time, but positive results can be on the way.

Relieving PMS pain.

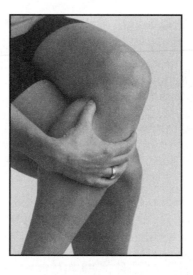

Locate SP-9 (Yin Tomb Spring) with your knee bent. Proceed to the inside center of the knee and move down toward your foot. This point can be located with legs crossed or uncrossed. When you hit soft, tender tissue in the crease of bone, that's it. Breathe slowly and deeply as you press firmly for one to two minutes. This point helps relieve abdominal pain, bloating, PMS, and painful periods. For additional acu-points, review Chapter 16, "Birthing Baby," and Chapter 17.

Ovarian Cysts and Uterine Fibroids: Double Trouble

Both of these are unwanted guests in your abdominal cavity. Ovarian cysts are caused by growing cells in the uterus (see the discussion on endometriosis earlier in this chapter), which attach to and penetrate the tough covering of the ovary and begin to multiply. These cells form a cyst—a closed pocket of tissue—and can collect a large amount of blood, growing to the size of an egg or grapefruit. They are often called chocolate cysts because the blood darkens as it collects, giving it the appearance of a piece of chocolate attached to the ovary. Some women do not even know they have cysts, while others feel the characteristic lower abdominal achiness and discomfort. Sudden or sharp pain may point to a rupture of the cyst. Twisted ovarian cysts produce intermittent pain and are usually removed if pain becomes persistent.

Uterine fibroids are benign (nonmalignant) tumors of muscle and connective tissue that develop within or are attached to the wall of the uterus. Fibroids usually appear in women older than age 20, and affect 15–20 percent of all women of reproductive age. For reasons not completely understood, uterine fibroids occur three to nine times more frequently in African-American women than Caucasian women.

Half of all women with fibroids never even know they have them, because there are no symptoms. The other half experience a wide range of complaints such as heavy and frequent menstrual bleeding, infertility, pain or bleeding with sexual intercourse, painful urination and bowel movements.

Acu-Points to Block the Bleeding

Many women who come to my practice are opting to use acupuncture and Oriental Medicine to stop the pain and excessive bleeding from fibroids and cysts. I make sure that they have been properly examined and diagnosed by their conventional physician to rule out any malignant growths. Over 30 percent of all hysterectomies (removal of the uterus) in the United States are done to remove uterine fibroids. Since these growths shrink after menopause, avoiding surgery is an option some women are choosing, and Oriental Medicine is a helpful partner.

To shrink the cysts or fibroids, acupuncture is often accompanied by herbal medicine or moxibustion (see Chapter 5, "Acupuncture—Tools of the Trade"). Cysts and fibroids vary in their oriental diagnosis according to your body's health and general well-being. According to traditional theory, emotional stress is the most common cause of abdominal masses. Anger and worry tend to slow down the flow of Qi and blood in the lower abdomen. Consumption of cold and greasy foods can also aggravate certain masses, and impair your own immune system. Your acu-pro

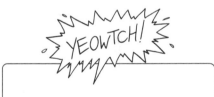

Harm Alarm

Ease off the estrogen. High estrogen birth control pills may increase the growth of uterine fibroids. Avoid oral contraceptives with high estrogen and seek alternatives.

will first determine what kind of characteristics your masses have, so a treatment plan can be created.

The traditional oriental classification of causes includes

➤ **Stuck Qi.** Masses seem to come and go, and it feels like you can move them; pain is present but has no fixed location; abdomen feels bloated.

➤ **Stuck Blood.** Pain is stabbing and has a fixed location, and the fibroids are not movable and feel hard.

➤ **Phlegm.** Masses feel soft and have a fixed location; usually the patient experiences no pain.

According to traditional Oriental Medicine the abnormally heavy bleeding is a symptom of a particular diagnostic pattern. Most women who exhibit this type of heavy bleeding usually show other symptoms that confirm a pattern of underlying weakness. This pattern may be seen with whatever type of abdominal mass they are dealing with. I find that Oriental Medicine works well to help build up the lost Qi, improving overall health while the specific symptoms are being reduced.

Easing the pain and excessive bleeding caused by abdominal masses.

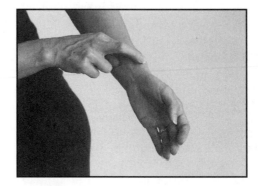

Locate LU-7 (Broken Sequence), which is about two-finger widths above the wrist crease on the side of your thumb. Hold this point with your index finger, taking easy, deep breaths for two to three minutes. Do both sides, together with KD-6 (see the next figure).

Easing the pain and excessive bleeding caused by abdominal masses.

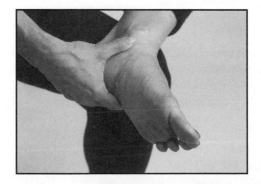

180

Locate KD-6 (Shining Sea) directly below the inside anklebone. Hold this point with your thumb or index finger, taking easy, deep breaths for two to three minutes. Do both sides, together with LU-7. These acu-points activate the channels specific to abdominal masses.

Bladder Infections: Say Goodbye to UTI

Bladder infections, also known as cystitis, are one of the most common conditions among women of all ages. According to a new study at the University of Washington School of Medicine, an estimated 7 million episodes of acute cystitis occur annually in the United States with an annual cost of $1 billion. The study further showed the term "honeymoon cystitis" is still accurate in that having sexual intercourse increases the risk of developing the condition. *Escherichia coli* (*E. coli*) bacteria found in fecal material is responsible for up to 90 percent of all urinary tract infections (UTI). Fecal-contaminated bacteria gains access to the bladder through the urethra.

Women are 30 times more likely to have cystitis than men due mostly to the different lengths of the urethra (women's urethras are just one-and-a-half inches long, while men have urethras about eight inches long). Men experience UTIs with obstructions like urinary stones or enlarged prostate. According to the National Bladder Foundation, an estimated 3 percent of girls and 1 percent of boys have UTIs by the age of 11. Among elderly women living in nursing homes or hospitalized, 20–50 percent will develop asymptomatic bacteriuria, which is a UTI without symptoms. The elderly and pregnant women are at risk for this type of UTI, which is symptom free but can still develop into serious kidney infections if left untreated.

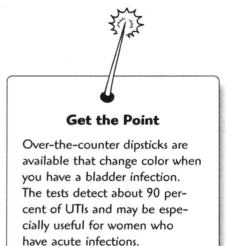

Get the Point

Over-the-counter dipsticks are available that change color when you have a bladder infection. The tests detect about 90 percent of UTIs and may be especially useful for women who have acute infections.

Risk Factors: Keeping an Eye on the UTI

As discussed, UTIs are extremely common. However, there are certain risk factors that appear to increase an individual's chances of developing the condition. They include

➤ A medical history of diabetes or sickle cell.

➤ Being an elderly woman who lives in a hospital or nursing home.

➤ Being a man over 65 years of age with prostate problems.

➤ Decreased estrogen amounts in postmenopausal women, which reduces *lactobacilli,* the body's normal infection-fighting microorganism.

➤ Sexual intercourse; the associated risk increases with frequency.

➤ Pregnancy; 4–10 percent of expectant women routinely found bacteria in the urine.

181

➤ Having a urinary catheter in place, especially longer than 30 days.

➤ Antibiotic use.

➤ Use of vaginal creams or other chemicals in the genital area.

Acu-Points: Concerning Your Burning

I get a great deal of satisfaction when I hear how acupuncture and Oriental Medicine have helped turn someone's life around who has been struggling with chronic bladder infections. The U.S. Census Bureau estimates that there will be a 12-percent increase in the number of bladder diseases over the next 15 years, with a dramatic 28-percent increase among women and men 40–59 years of age. Oriental Medicine can help us understand why this may be happening when we look at the characteristic causes of UTIs. They include

➤ **External dampness.** This condition may arise from sitting in wet grass, wearing a wet bathing suit, or living in a damp environment.

➤ **Diet.** Eating excessive amounts of sugar, dairy, and greasy or spicy foods can cause UTIs.

➤ **Excessive sexual activity.** A lot of sexual activity increases exposure to bacteria and weakens lower-body Qi (Kidney Qi).

➤ **Age.** As your Qi weakens with age, your immune system struggles to fight off illness; look for dripping or difficult urination.

➤ **Emotional stress.** Anger, frustration, and resentment cause Qi to stagnate, while chronic anxiety, grief, or sadness weaken the body and build up heat often felt in the chest and lower abdomen.

➤ **Trauma or surgery.** Excessive lifting of heavy objects injures the low back and stagnates Qi in the abdominal region. Likewise, women who have had surgery, such as a hysterectomy, often suffer from recurrent cystitis.

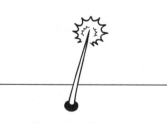

Get the Point

Drink cranberry juice! In a recent Israeli study, drinking 1½ cups of cranberry juice a day for six months helped keep 85 percent of elderly women bacteria free. Cranberry juice and blueberries prevent *E. coli* bacteria from sticking to cells of the urinary tract, so they can't stay around to cause trouble.

I have found that acupuncture is a great treatment for bladder infections, whether they are chronic or acute. Often an antibiotic can be avoided if you get to your acu-pro in time. I suggest staying in close communication with your physician so that you can be sure your treatments are effective. Women who come in for chronic cystitis are particularly pleased when the cycle of pain and burning is over.

Typically, I will use acupuncture and prescribe an herbal formula for their condition and overall health. I have also given them a second herbal prescription if acute symptoms arise. Diet and stress management are quite important for continuous relief. Acupressure and regular exercise are an effective tag team for home care. Common herbs for this condition include Bian Xu, Che Qian Zi, Mu Tong, and Fu Ling. A qualified herbalist will be able to create an individualized approach customized to your needs.

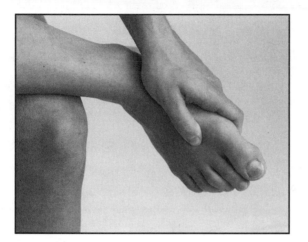

Treating bladder infections.

Locate LIV-3 (Great Pouring), which is in the middle of the webbing between the big toe and the second toe. Using your thumb, press firmly into the sorest spot for one or two minutes. Breathe deeply, repeating two to four times per session. Additional acupoints that can affect the bladder include SP-6 (see Chapter 16) and SP-99 (discussed in this chapter).

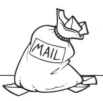

Mailbag

Karen was 32 years of age and suffered since high school from chronic bladder infections. She had severe PMS and a bladder infection almost every month. She had just gotten married and her chronic cystitis was affecting her marriage, as well as work and an active sports life. We initially used acupuncture, which quickly gave her relief from the burning and urgency. After combining weekly acupuncture visits with Chinese herbs and dietary changes such as reducing sugars, caffeine, and most alcohol, Karen was able to stay off antibiotics, increase her sports activity, cut back on acupuncture visits, and have a satisfying relationship with her new husband.

One of the greatest joys I get out of being in practice is to hear how women have changed some of the conditions that they experienced as limitations in their life and turn them around with new insight and inspiration. I'm grateful to have been a part of the assistance they used in order to feel more balanced and in control. Keep turning those pages to find out the options available for the numerous digestive complaints that can often make mealtime a nightmare.

The Least You Need to Know

➤ Annually, about 12 million women are diagnosed with endometriosis. The symptoms are often ignored as being part of menstrual discomfort.

➤ Acupuncture can regulate your cycle and reduce endometriosis pain and dysfunction.

➤ Abnormal uterine bleeding from fibroids and ovarian cysts can be greatly relieved by Oriental Medicine.

➤ Bladder infections get the boot with acu-points.

Chapter 19

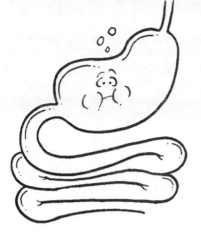

Gastrointestinal Conditions—A Glitch in Your Gut

In This Chapter

➤ Regulate the unruly movements of irritable bowel syndrome

➤ Clear your congested colon of constipation

➤ Slow down determined diarrhea

➤ Knock down nagging nausea

We're definitely into a topic that no one discusses: the glitches in your gut. It just is not polite conversation to describe your bothersome bowel habits to your friends and family. Yet these conditions, if left untreated, go a long way in determining your quality of life. Do you look for the location of the closest restroom wherever you go? How many times have you turned down invitations to go out boating, hiking, or for dinner because of how you digest food?

You are not alone. Over 60 million Americans (one in four) suffer from a variety of uncomfortable and often embarrassing gastrointestinal (GI) complaints. According to Dr. William Chey, medical director of the Konar Center for Digestive and Liver Disease, digestive disorders are the number one reason for absenteeism due to illness among female workers. All you have to do is look at the shelves of any corner drugstore to know how prevalent GI problems are in our society. Keep turning these pages, and I'll give you news and insights that you can swallow and digest.

Irritable Bowel Syndrome: A Moving Experience

Irritable bowel syndrome, or IBS, is the most common digestive condition in the United States, affecting one in five adults. Twice as many are women than men. The condition occurs when the normal rhythm of your colon becomes irregular, typically leaving you experiencing diarrhea, cramping abdominal pain, bloating, constipation, or nausea. Pockets of trapped intestinal gas can cause pain, especially after eating, and are often temporarily relieved by bowel movements. Victims may dread mealtime due to the anticipated discomfort afterward.

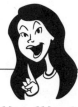

Wise Words

The November 11, 1999, issue of *The Journal of the American Medical Association* reported that Chinese herbal medicine appears to significantly alleviate symptoms of irritable bowel syndrome. Read all about it and see your acu-pro!

Common triggers of IBS include stress, food intolerances (such as high fat content), and hormonal changes. Your physician may schedule tests such as a proctosigmoidoscopy to examine the inside lining of the bowel to rule out conditions such as Crohn's disease, diverticulitis, lactose intolerance, and ulcerative colitis. There are few well-controlled studies that demonstrate the benefit of any one medication.

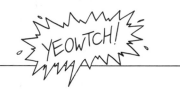

Harm Alarm

Dairy products, wheat bran, wheat products, caffeine, alcohol, sorbitol-containing chewing gums and sodas, nuts, fatty foods, chocolate, and fried foods—these produce mucus and block nutrient absorption. Cut them out of your diet if at all possible.

Acu-Points for Bothersome Bowels

I've helped many patients return to a more normal life through Oriental Medicine. In addition to working out an acupressure and acupuncture plan, I also help my patients address lifestyle habits, such as diet and stress management. Typical treatment lasts for several months, with acupuncture sessions spreading farther apart as your condition stabilizes and your own self-care becomes more effective. I also recommend that my patients begin taking acidophilus and bifidus supplements. These are the naturally occurring bacteria that are supposed to be in your intestines, but frequently are depleted with diarrhea. Adding fruit and fiber, plus whole grains like brown rice, can help stabilize your colon and reduce painful spasms.

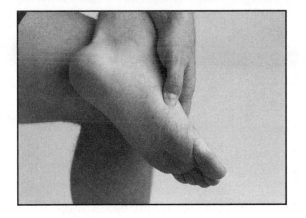

Alleviating bowel problems.

Locate SP-4 (Grandfather's Grandson) on the inside of the foot, one-finger width before the first joint of the big toe. Press with one or two thumbs directly into the side of the foot for one or two minutes. Repeat several times on each foot to help with stomachache, nausea, and bloating. Additional IBS acu-points include ST-36, PC-6, and SP-6 (see Chapter 16, "Birthing Baby").

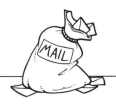

Mailbag

Bill led a busy life as a television producer, college professor, and father. His day was made even more challenging by severe abdominal cramps, foul intestinal gas, and the need to move his bowels about five times per day. I used acupuncture therapy to calm the colon spasms, and reduce the pain and frequent bowel movements. Supplements of probiotics such as acidophilus, bifidus, and Chinese herbs further helped stabilize his colon, adding energy and free time to his day. He cut dairy and wheat out of his diet. Now he eats without anxiety.

Constipation: Ready, Set, No Go!

Your digestive system is amazing and efficient … most of the time. All your food and drinks are processed by flowing through more than 30 feet of intestines. In a matter of a few hours, nutrients are loaded into your bloodstream, while the waste material

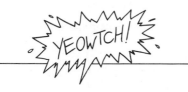

is separated and stored temporarily in your colon. Excess water that your body cannot use elsewhere is removed, and when you feel the urge to purge, you have a bowel movement (or BM, as my mother so politely called it!).

What if the urge never comes knocking, is infrequent, or it's painful and difficult to pass the waste material (or stool)? That is what commonly is called constipation. The longer your stool sits in the colon, the more water keeps getting pulled out, making it dryer and harder and even more difficult to pass.

Constipation is a frequent GI complaint, especially among women, children, and those over age 65. Again, we don't talk about it, but it can lead to various maladies, including bad breath, body odor, depression, headaches, hemorrhoids, indigestion, insomnia, gas, and fatigue.

Harm Alarm

Bowel cancer is the second-most frequent cancer among men over 50 (lung cancer is first). You'll notice sudden changes in bowel habits (constipation or diarrhea), blood in the stool, or abdominal pain. Make an appointment with your physician if you have any suspicions.

Constipation most often is a result of insufficient fiber and fluids. Some medications, such as painkillers and antidepressants, as well as iron supplements, can cause constipation.

Acu-Pros Hasten to Relieve Constipation

Believe it or not, the frequency and quantity of bowel movements differ from culture to culture. According to *Don't Forget Fiber in Your Diet,* rural African adults pass 400–500 grams of stool daily, while the typical westerner passes about 80–120 grams. The time it takes for food and drink to move through your bowels determines how often you have to "go." In rural Africa, transit time is one-and-a-half days, while people in western societies average three days. I believe that if you are eating and drinking regularly, a daily bowel movement is a reasonable expectation.

Oriental Medicine categorizes constipation by your individual overall health. For instance, deficient yin symptoms include dry stools, thirst, dry mouth and throat (especially in the evenings), sore back and knees, night sweats, dizziness, and ringing in the ears. Effective treatments are available for this and other forms of constipation. It's not unusual for patients to have overused laxatives in order to move their bowels. I generally begin treatments of acupuncture, lifestyle and nutritional counseling, perhaps herbal medicine to lubricate the bowel, stop intestinal spasms or atrophy and gradually back off the laxatives.

Self-abdominal massages such as those we described in Chapter 14, "Childhood Conditions—Pass the Owner's Manual," for colic are helpful to awaken and regulate your bowels.

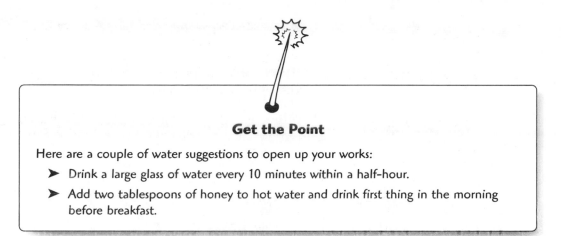

Get the Point

Here are a couple of water suggestions to open up your works:

➤ Drink a large glass of water every 10 minutes within a half-hour.

➤ Add two tablespoons of honey to hot water and drink first thing in the morning before breakfast.

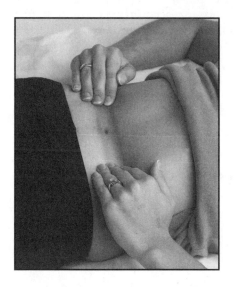

Place your palms on both sides of the abdomen and gently stretch the colon by applying even and gradual pressure to the sides at the same time. Combine this with the colic massage discussed in Chapter 14 and repeat one to two times per day.

Diarrhea: Runs for Your Life!

Diarrhea involves bowel movements that are loose and watery. About 60–90 percent of stool weight consists of water, but when the water content goes too high, you know it. Abdominal pain and cramping, a sense of urgency to have a bowel movement, and sometimes nausea or vomiting are the clues you'll get if you have mild diarrhea.

Severe diarrhea may be a sign of serious illness and may be accompanied by blood, mucus, or undigested food in your stool, weight loss, or fever. Contact your health-care provider promptly if these severe symptoms persist longer than 24 hours. Losing all this fluid can deplete much-needed water and salts that your body needs to function. Keep drinking water to replace lost fluids.

189

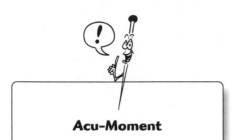

Acu-Points to Slow the Flow

People around the world have been dealing with diarrhea for centuries. Oriental Medicine has developed effective strategies to treat acute or chronic diarrhea. A mild case of diarrhea helps your body clean out toxins and bacteria, and is of little concern for the first two days. However, I see patients who have continual loose stools that disrupt their lives and who need safe and effective solutions for their conditions.

I find that irregular diet, emotional stress, and overwork are frequently at the root of chronic diarrhea. After our initial exam, your total condition will be taken into account as a comprehensive treatment plan is designed for you. I use acupuncture, nutrition, and Qi Gong meditation to slow the flow. Chinese herbs can also be used to treat underlying conditions that lead to poor overall health and loose stools. Qi Gong meditations such as standing facing a beautiful forest, pond, or stream while you breathe deeply in through your nose imagining the peacefulness and majesty of nature flowing into you and exhaling all the unwanted tension or toxins out of your mouth are a great way to help with the excess worry and stress that often accompany diarrhea. Depending on the diagnosis, herbs such as Bai Tou Weng, Huang Lian, Fu Ling, and Bai Zhu will be used to reduce the spasms in your colon and regain optimal health for preventative care of your digestive tract.

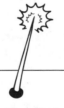

Get the Point

An estimated 30–50 percent of endurance runners experience cramping, gas, nausea, and diarrhea known as runner's trots. Vigorous exercise reduces the blood to the intestines, and the up-and-down mechanical stress causes untimely run-ins.

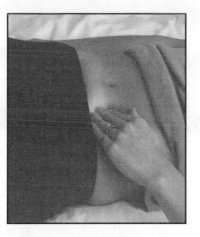

Dealing with diarrhea.

Locate SP-15 (Big Horizontal), which is three-finger width on either side of your navel. Rest your palms on your belly, bend your fingers, and press deeply into the abdomen for one to two minutes. Close your eyes and breathe deeply. Relax. This point helps diarrhea or constipation.

Indigestion: It's Easy to Be Queasy

Don't you just hate eating a meal and being reminded of it for several hours afterward? The little candy mints aren't enough to stop the heartburn, gas, abdominal pain, and bloated or nauseous feeling that indigestion brings our way. Indigestion seems to be growing as a condition; I know I see it more frequently in the office. Perhaps our modern lifestyle has something to do with it.

Tips to End Indigestion

Try working in a few of these tips and see if your digestion improves. If it does, keep it going.

➤ **Chew with your mouth closed.** Swallowing air or talking while eating can make it worse.

➤ **Chew food till it's close to liquid form.** This makes your stomach's job easier, and foods need the enzymes in your saliva to digest properly.

➤ **Hold the drinks.** Drinking fluids, especially cold sodas or ice water, dilutes stomach enzymes.

➤ **Relax and eat slowly.** Stress, anxiety, and worry can disrupt the digestive mechanism.

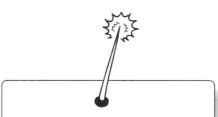

Get the Point

You need hydrochloric acid (HCL) to digest food. Is your stomach making enough? Swallow a tablespoon of lemon juice or vinegar (both are loaded with HCL). If your indigestion goes away, you need more acid in your diet. If it's worse, you've got *too* much acid in the stomach.

191

➤ **Take a seat.** Enjoying your meal while seated helps your body focus on digestion. Eating while standing or driving can increase indigestion.

➤ **Cut out the aggravators.** Reduce or eliminate alcohol, vinegar, caffeine, and refined, junk, spicy, or greasy foods, which can trigger indigestion.

Acu-Points: Get a Break from Your Stomachache

I see more indigestion every year as our lives race forward. Acu-point stimulation can significantly decrease your symptoms, especially if combined with the lifestyle and eating-habit changes outlined earlier in this chapter.

Easing indigestion.

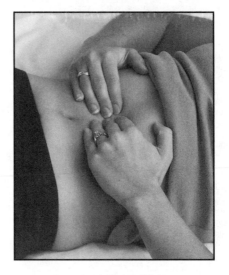

Locate CV-12 (Middle Cavity), which is four-finger widths directly above your navel. Press into this point firmly for one to two minutes, followed by deep breathing as you slowly rub and massage the point in a clockwise direction. This point aids in stomachaches, nausea, and gastritis.

Eating is such a basic function of life that when it's disrupted you notice it on every level. The solutions you've just read about will help harmonize the stomach and colon with the use of Oriental techniques. We go from the extreme inside of the body conditions to the farthest outside possible: the skin.

The Least You Need to Know

➤ Acu-points can greatly reduce the discomfort of IBS.

➤ Constipation can be cut short by adding plenty of fluids, fiber, and exercise throughout each day.

➤ Colon massage and stretching help stuck intestines move right along.

➤ Keep drinking water to avoid dehydration during diarrhea.

➤ Sit down, slow down, and chew your food well to avoid heartburn and indigestion.

Chapter 20

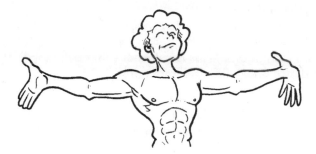

Skin—The Purpose of the Surface

In This Chapter

➤ Learn how your skin reflects your overall health

➤ Itchy and embarrassing eczema takes an exit with Oriental Medicine

➤ Wave bye-bye to worry lines and crow's-feet with an acu-point facelift

---

Your skin is the largest organ you've got. It envelops your body in a waterproof protective covering that will take all kinds of abuse from birth through midlife crisis. Is there a price to pay? You bet. According to traditional oriental theory, your skin reflects the inner workings of your body and spirit. Organs like the stomach, lungs, and bowels can greatly affect the texture, tone, and glow of your skin. Keep reading to learn some tips for stunning skin.

Eczema: Ditch the Itch

Eczema is also known as atopic dermatitis and affects between 3 and 7 percent of our population. In more than 70 percent of patients, it runs in the family. The skin typically becomes dry, flaking, scaling, and thickening. It also often changes color, and itching can develop.

Eczema occurs most often on the face, wrists, elbows, and knees, but it is not limited to those areas. You're likely to discover it on your newborn baby or infant, although many children outgrow it before their second birthdays. If they do not, they are likely to be chronic sufferers with distinctive thickened brownish-gray skin where the outbreaks frequently occur.

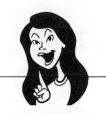

Wise Words

Food allergies can escalate eczema. Common culprits that often contribute to eczema include wheat, dairy, sugar, eggs, processed foods, peanuts, strawberries, shrimp, and fried foods. Watch what your child eats and observe his or her symptoms for 24 hours to see if there's a connection.

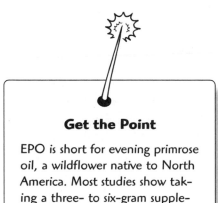

Get the Point

EPO is short for evening primrose oil, a wildflower native to North America. Most studies show taking a three- to six-gram supplement of EPO a day for at least three months can have a positive effect on eczema.

Asthma and allergies seem to be a troublesome twosome that may accompany your eczema. The pattern I often see is an infant who develops or is born with eczema and is diagnosed with allergic asthma by the time he or she is four or five years old. If you or your child have eczema, please refer to Chapter 14, "Childhood Conditions—Pass the Owner's Manual," for guidance on asthma treatment and prevention.

When you think of the skin as showing us what's going on inside, you will treat eczema with a total health perspective and increase your chances for a successful outcome.

Oriental Medicine Makes the Connection

Today we benefit from the meticulous observations and connections made by Chinese doctors over 2,000 years ago. Eastern practitioners have already developed treatment strategies for the close relationship between the lungs and your skin that is born out in today's Western medical journals.

Wind-heat eczema is characterized by skin lesions that are dry, red, itchy, and move around all over your body. With damp-heat eczema, you'll find skin lesions that are moist, oozing fluid, and red, and the itchiness is located in specific locations like the forearms or legs. Which one of these do you recognize for yourself or your child?

Acupuncture can significantly reduce the itching and eruptions of eczema. I will frequently employ the use of nutrition to weed out food allergies and herbs to keep the whole body balanced. Since most of these patients have a family history of eczema or allergies, we work to balance or correct deep-seated deficiencies in your overall health. Be patient—the results are worth it.

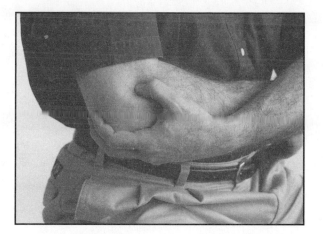

Easing the discomfort of eczema.

Locate LI-11 (Crooked Pool); with the arm bent at the elbow, the acu-point is on the outside of the elbow, halfway between the elbow crease and bone that sticks out on the side. Press for one to two minutes, breathing deeply, or rub gently on an infant. This acu-point will reduce itchiness and redness from wind-heat eczema. Additional acu-points that can alleviate eczema include Ding Chuan, LU-1 (Chapter 12, "Respiration—A Breath of Fresh Air"), ST-36, and LI-4 (Chapter 16, "Birthing Baby").

Facelifts: An Uplifting Experience

When the energy required to weather life's ups and downs begins to show on your face, what do you do? According to the Mayo Clinic Women's Health Source, at least 80,000 people in 1999 decided to have a facelift (rhytidectomy). Facelifts are the fourth-most common elective procedure behind liposuction, breast augmentation, and eyelid surgery, according to the American Society of Plastic and Reconstructive Surgeons. Women had more than 90 percent of the facelifts performed in 1999. While many of them were done to push back the clock, some facelifts are performed due to diseases, disfigurement, or traumas that emotionally as well as physically scar the individual.

Most facelifts are performed under local anesthesia and a sedative that makes you drowsy. Some surgeons perform general anesthesia so that you'll sleep through the operation. Incisions are made on either side of your face from inside the hairline. Loose skin is pulled up and back, and the excess is cut away. Experts suggest you will be up and about in a day or two, and recovery usually takes up to two weeks due to bruising and swelling. The average cost of a facelift in America is approximately $4,500, with an additional $1,000 for anesthesia.

> **YEOWTCH!**
>
> **Harm Alarm**
>
> Quit smoking ... before you get a facelift. Smoking has an adverse effect on the skin, due to nicotine contracting blood flow, and greatly increases your risk of scarring and complications with a surgical facelift.

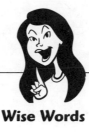

Wise Words

Facelift Facts:

➤ Ninety-nine percent of all cosmetic surgeries are performed on women.

➤ Eighty-one percent of patients are between the ages of 35 and 64; 51 percent are between 51 and 64.

➤ Average cost is $4,500 plus $1,000 for anesthesia.

➤ Benefits last 10 years for women in their 40s; only 5 years for women in their 60s.

Source: The American Society of Plastic and Reconstructive Surgery

Acu-Facelift

Acu-points circulate much-needed blood and vital Qi throughout our bodies, including the face. Just as the rest of your skin can improve with Oriental Medicine, so can your looks. While these procedures are not performed as much as those designed to treat, say, backaches or asthma, I've had some success with them and want to share them with you as an option for your skin care.

Here's how I perform acupuncture for healthy facial skin and skin tone. I insert tiny 3–6 millimeter needles into worry lines, crow's-feet, and smile lines to bring much-needed circulation to the sagging, malnourished skin. Once I remove the needles, a facial massage is employed. Some practitioners use herbs and oils on the skin that enhance healing. I teach patients to do their own facial massage, allowing more frequent stimulation and helping patients become more involved in the healing process.

I combine this with regular needle acupuncture to treat the patient's overall health, because the skin reflects it all. I also make some nutritional recommendations, including taking the supplement Coenzyme Q10, which is a powerful antioxidant.

Acu-points cannot trim or suck the fat from around your neck. They can, however, fill in many of the lines and wrinkles in your face and bring a glow of vitality to your smile. There are no side effects or recovery time, and you get the additional benefit of feeling good all over. Check with your acu-pro to make sure he or she has experience in this specialized area of Oriental Medicine.

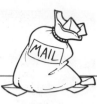

Mailbag

Sandy had been recently divorced and was making all the exercise, nutritional habits, and career moves to make a new life for herself. She felt self-conscious about the crows' feet wrinkles that were on the outside corners of her eyes. To her they represented the years of worry and anguish that she left behind with her divorce. They were not anything that she thought about having surgery for, but would still like to get rid of them. I began to use tiny facial acupuncture needles on her wrinkles that are so small I need tweezers to put them in. They are also painless and go in the end of the wrinkles to stimulate blood flow. Following the treatments her face felt a little tighter, until after her twelfth treatment she was pleased with the retreating wrinkles and was off to enjoy a new life. I've not seen her since, but I'm sure that the happiness and beauty she created and fostered on her inside have continued to shine and be noticeable to all on the outside.

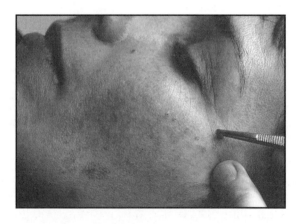

Tiny 3–6-millimeter needles are held with tweezers and inserted into the ends and middle of wrinkles. The needle insertion is followed by approximately 30 minutes of relaxation.

The red, itchy patches of eczema and the equally unwanted wrinkles of our face can be greatly alleviated with the tools of Oriental Medicine. Nothing to stress about, which brings me to the next chapter, "Stress—Notions and Emotions." This is a must-read chapter for anyone out in today's world of fast-paced deals and drive-through meals.

A facial massage and acu-point treatment are given following your acupuncture. Relax and enjoy.

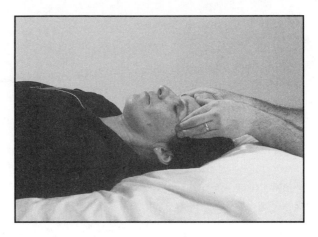

The Least You Need to Know

➤ The skin is your largest organ and reflects the condition of your overall health.

➤ Eczema is usually hereditary, often along with a family history of asthma.

➤ Oriental Medicine can clean your skin of itchy lesions and improve your overall health.

➤ Eighty thousand people (90 percent of them women) had facelifts in 1999.

➤ An acu-facelift can help fill up wrinkles and smile lines, but will not clear away neck fat or sagging jowls.

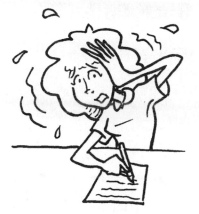

Chapter 21

Stress—Notions and Emotions

In This Chapter

➤ Use acu-points to wring the worry from your mind

➤ Relaxing and revitalizing Qi Gong brings balance and peace to your everyday life

➤ Lifting the spirits of depression with Oriental Medicine

➤ Calm anxious nerves with time-tested acu-points and herbs

Feeling a little stressed? It seems that most of us experience some form of stress throughout the day. Stress is your body's reaction to external factors, either physical or emotional. How it affects us depends on the amount of stress, the length of time we're under the gun, and our capacity to handle the load. With our lives in high gear, and multitasking a necessity, it's no wonder that some days it can all seem too much!

The World Health Organization lists acupuncture as a suitable treatment for anxiety and depression. In this chapter, you will learn how working with your acu-pro and other health professionals can ease your emotional burden. My patients have found a real release from stress and worry using acu-points and medical Qi Gong breathing exercises.

You'll learn how to "check in" with yourself to discover if your normal level of stress is becoming a potential anxiety or depression concern. Mental and emotional challenges *are* real. I see them as a growing component of many of my patients' overall health imbalances. Oriental medicine and acu-points are valuable partners in your path for peace of mind. Now, take a slow deep breath, in through the nose, exhale with an audible sigh … aaahhh.

Stress: Burning the Candle at Both Ends

Your workload has doubled since the layoffs at your place of employment, both your toddlers are home sick from school, your town leaf pickup is in two days, and you forgot your mother's birthday. As you feel your heart pound, your blood pressure rises, muscles tense, and the pupils of your eyes open wider. Guess what? You're stressed. It's the old fight-or-flight reaction: Should I stay on or should I go?

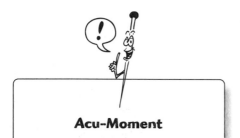

Acu-Moment

Hans Selye, M.D., Ph.D., is internationally recognized as the father of the study of stress. In 1936, he popularized the term **stress** to identify the nonspecific and adverse reaction that any creature experiences when placed under too much demand.

According to Richard Earle, Ph.D. at the Canadian Institute of Stress, American corporate life has certainly contributed to our stress levels. Dr. Earle states that during the last 10 years in America, half of all corporations have restructured, over 90,000 have been acquired or merged, 240,000 have downsized, and half a million U.S. companies have failed. This unstable business environment undoubtedly contributes to continuing pressure and diminished coping ability among working Americans, which in turn creates feelings of insecurity and inadequacy. "There's a lot going on, and I can't handle it," is a common complaint. We just can't keep up with the workload. Combine this with the commitment and responsibilities of being a spouse and/or parent. Forget it!

Most of us can rally for short-term or acute stressful situations. It's when the pressure stays on for extended periods of time that a condition is created that is harder to shake.

Continued stress can weaken your body's immune system. Researchers at The Children's Hospital of Pittsburgh found a biological component that links stress to the common cold.

The Stress Show: Your Price of Admission

Stress wreaks havoc on your body, and its effects can disrupt any number of systems. Here's a list of typical signs and symptoms of too much stress.

Physical Symptoms

- ➤ Headache
- ➤ Fatigue
- ➤ Back pain
- ➤ Neck pain

- ➤ Loss of appetite
- ➤ Overeating or binge eating
- ➤ High blood pressure
- ➤ Digestive changes

Mental/Emotional Symptoms

➤ Tension

➤ Anxiety

➤ Depression

➤ Anger

➤ Antisocial behavior

➤ Pessimism

➤ Cynicism

➤ Difficulty concentrating

Had Enough? Let Go of Stress

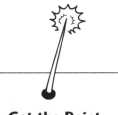

Stress is part of almost every patient's list of concerns. How much it affects his or her overall health depends on the mind/body reaction. I have successfully treated acute stress when symptoms are sparked by a job change or moving to a new town. With chronic stress, your body has already been adapting to the constant state of tension.

You probably have physical and emotional symptoms to untangle. The beauty of Oriental Medicine is that all your individual feelings and symptoms can be used to discover your Qi imbalances. For instance, the most common form of stress I see is called stagnation of liver Qi, in Oriental Medical terms. This means that Qi is stuck in your body, and the symptoms that you have are associated with the liver Qi channel or organ in oriental pathology.

The typical pattern of stress would include moodiness, irritability, frustration, annoyance, belching, irregular menstrual periods, tight feeling in the chest, and fatigue. In most cases, acupuncture treatments and home acupressure will help bring you back on course. Herbs, proper nutrition, exercise, and medical Qi Gong may be added to suit the individual needs of the patient. Dealing with the source of the stress is paramount to feeling better in the long term. Acu-points provide the window of opportunity to keep stress at arm's length instead of in your face so that you can continue healing.

> **Get the Point**
>
> Ears ... the window to your soul? As you read in Chapter 9, "Pain Below the Belt," your ear acu-points lead to your whole body. An acu-ear treatment will strike out at your stress. Close your eyes and hold both earlobes between your thumbs and index fingers. Gently squeeze while breathing slowly and deeply. Move up and over your ear, lightly pinching as you go. Gently cup your ears in your hand and slowly stretch them by moving forward and backward. Cover them with cupped hands and breathe slowly in and out for 30 seconds. Closing your eyes also shuts out distractions and helps you relax.

Oriental nutritional recommendations borrow much from the herbal culture. Both, to be the most effective, are individually prescribed by a qualified practitioner that examines and balances your whole system. If you had been experiencing chronic stress that resulted in erratic moods, insomnia that began after early waking, a red- to scarlet-tipped tongue, and increased thirst, an Oriental Medical diagnosis of deficient

203

heart yin would be appropriate. To help you properly nourish and balance your body I might suggest adding bitter gourd, crab apple, muskmelon, watermelon, adzuki bean, or persimmon to your diet. Commonly used Chinese herbs for this stage of stress include Bai Zi Ren, Fu Shen, He Huan Pi, and Yuan Zi. Check with your acu-pro to make sure you're making the right choice for yourself.

Stopping stress.

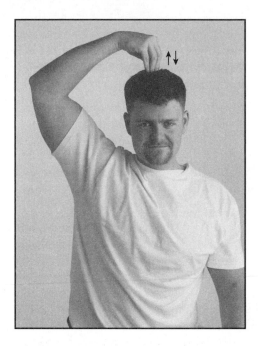

Locate GV-20 (Hundred Meetings), which is found by following a line from the tip of your ears to midpoint on the top of your head. With relaxed, bent fingers, tap the point and surrounding area lightly while breathing deeply. To further help stagnant liver Qi, whisper the word "sha" as you exhale. This is an ancient Chinese healing sound to help release tension and stress.

Worry: Who, Me?

I've thought about it a hundred times and I still can't make a choice. My dreams, both during the day and at night, are filled with shifting scenarios and made-up conversations. Do I have anything to worry about?

We worry about our jobs, health, children, and the cost of groceries. The word "worry" is originally from a prehistoric German word which meant "to strangle." Worrying, as you know, puts a stranglehold on your mind and body as you churn ideas around all day. Worry cuts off other ideas that might be more useful, if only they could crowd their way into the narrowing passageway of your thoughts.

Work worries frequently wander through our minds. Christina Malachi and Michael Letter, authors of *The Truth About Burnout* (Jossey-Bass, 1997), have identified six areas of worry in the workplace: workload, control, reward, community, fairness, and values. The authors feel that if these six areas are balanced at your job, you are less likely to develop into a worry warrior.

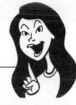

Wise Words

Discover your worry gap by rating yourself in two areas. On a scale from 0 (no biggie) to 10 (major problem):

➤ What's your worry level?

➤ How important is this thing, anyway?

If you are jamming an 8 worry level into a 2 situation, rethink your investment of time and energy.

Acu-Pros Relieve the Worry Wart

Worry is listed as one of the pathogenic emotions that can injure your body over time. As you've read, worry originally meant "to strangle," and it certainly can strangle your Qi to stagnation. According to Oriental Medical theory, this can affect your lungs and digestion. Neck and shoulders get tense and painful. If worry has injured your lungs, you may feel breathlessness, a dryness in your throat, and an uncomfortable stifling feeling in your chest. Worry can also cause poor digestion, including abdominal pain, bloating, fatigue, and decreased appetite. I often see poor concentration and memory as well.

By the fourth century C.E., the Chinese had discovered that if certain emotions were experienced during a prolonged period of time, the body could be injured. *Yellow Emperor's Classic of Internal Medicine* lists these correspondences:

➤ Anger—Liver

➤ Joy—Heart

➤ Worry—Spleen and lungs

➤ Pensiveness—Spleen

➤ Sadness—Lungs and heart

➤ Fear—Kidneys

➤ Shock—Kidneys and heart

I have found that Oriental Medicine helps in recovery from the effects of our worrying. Getting to the root of the worry is important, and taking care of your body will give you a chance to be healthy during your search. Acupuncture, moxibustion, and herbs can help ease your mind and wipe away worry, allowing your Qi to properly flow and nourish you. According to Oriental Medical theory, when your system is deprived of smooth flowing Qi, imbalances begin to appear as your body tries to continually compensate in order to regain harmony. Acupuncture helps move the Qi along, which will give a feeling of pressure being released, while herbs and proper nutrition will sustain and fuel your body's continued efforts to fully heal. The break in the action reminds patients of what it can feel like to end the worry cycle.

Wiping out worry.

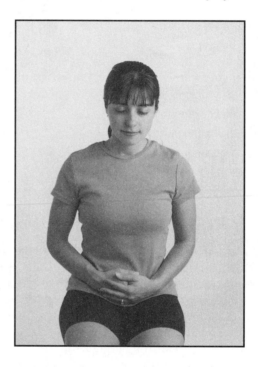

Sit or lie down in a supported position with your eyes closed. Imagine your spleen (located behind your stomach). Using your imagination, inhale deeply and see a yellow mist coat your spleen inside and out, as you slowly exhale and say the word "who" in an audible whisper. Imagine all the toxins and tension leaving your digestive system. These are the medical Qi Gong healing sounds and colors for your spleen. Repeat two to three times and enjoy!

Depression: Leaving the Black Hole Behind

Depression affects your whole body, from your nervous system and moods to the way you eat, sleep, and feel about yourself. Depression, in some form or other, affects 20 percent of all women, 10 percent of all men, and 5 percent of all adolescents worldwide. It's the most common emotional condition in the U.S., with more than 11 million Ameri-cans struggling to deal with it each year.

Although depression is two to four times more common in women than men, Dr. William Pollack of the Center for Men at McLean Hospital in Boston believes men's depression is extremely underdiagnosed. Each year, as many as 15 percent of people with depression commit suicide, most of whom are men.

The causes of depression are not fully understood. Heredity does play a key role; 50 percent of people who experience recurrent episodes of depression have one or both parents who have also experienced depression.

Depression Checklist: Are You at Risk?

There are many forms of depression. If you suffer from five or more of the following symptoms for at least a two-week period, I advise you to see your healthcare professional:

➤ Persistent sadness, pessimism

➤ Feelings of guilt, worthlessness, hopelessness

➤ Loss of interest or pleasure in ordinary activities, including intercourse

➤ Decreased energy, fatigue

➤ Insomnia, oversleeping, or early morning waking

➤ Difficulty concentrating and poor memory

➤ Loss of appetite, weight gain or loss

➤ Anxiety, irritability

➤ Suicidal thoughts

➤ Excessive crying

➤ Chronic aches and pains that don't respond to treatment

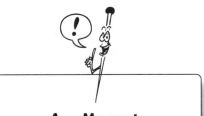

Acu-Moment

Seasonal affective disorder, or SAD, is experienced during the winter months when the days are shorter and darker. This type of depression is thought to be two to three times more prevalent in women than men and occurs more frequently in the Northern Hemisphere.

In children, the warning signs are

➤ Insomnia, fatigue, headache, stomachache, and dizziness

➤ Weight loss

➤ Apathy, social withdrawal

➤ Drug or alcohol abuse

➤ Drop in school performance

➤ Isolation from family and friends

Lifting Your Spirits with Acu-Points

Since there are many forms of depression, Oriental Medicine is well equipped to take your individual diagnosis and symptoms of overall health and find a treatment plan to help you out of the hole. My patients are often being seen simultaneously by psychiatrists, physiologists, or licensed social workers. I've found communication and involvement of the whole healing team the most beneficial for the patient's condition. I want to make sure my patients are getting all the help they need.

One of the most common diagnoses in traditional Oriental Medicine is heart-blood deficiency. As you can tell by the name, this condition deals with issues concerning the heart organ or channel. These issues are usually emotional. Blood deficiency implies an energetic weakness. This usually presents itself as palpitations, insomnia, poor memory, dizziness, jumpiness, dull complexion, confusion, and lack of concentration.

Our strategy includes nourishing the body with foods that are high in complex carbohydrates and protein. These contain essential nutrients to feed your brain. Acupuncture, moxibustion, and herbal medicine have been effective in clearing the mind, restoring good sleep, and bringing energy and centeredness into your being. Suan Zao Ren, Bai Zi Ren, Mu Li, Long Gu, and Dan Shen are just a few of the herbs that may be used in your formula.

I also recommend consistent, vigorous exercise, which produces those natural painkillers, endorphins and enkephalins. Both make you feel good. Depression can come and go instantly or over a period of weeks, months, or years. Using Oriental Medicine nourishes your body and mind and encourages your system to heal.

Defeating depression.

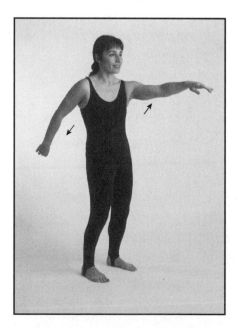

Stand or sit in an armless chair. While deeply breathing, slowly begin to swing your arms (either together or one in front while the other swings to the back). Close your eyes, relax, and think of a joyous time in your life filled with friends, laughter, and love. Gradually swing your arms higher and higher, but stopping before you're above the shoulder level. Let a smile come across your face as you gently slow your arms down and lower them until they are at your sides again. This Qi Gong exercise takes about five to ten minutes and is designed to open the heart and lung channels, oxygenating your blood and clearing your head.

Anxiety: A New Dimension in Apprehension

Most of us have felt anxious at one time or another. You tend to feel the characteristic adrenaline rush through your bloodstream as your heart rate quickens; breathing becomes shallow and rapid, muscles tense, sugar is released by your liver, and your mind goes on full alert. You are ready for action!

But what if there is no action or danger to tackle? When these symptoms are not connected to an identifiable threat or last longer than is warranted, then it's called an anxiety disorder. Your fight-or-flight response is geared to go at the wrong time.

There are several recognized anxiety disorders, including

➤ **Phobias.** Fear of specific situations (for example, insects, confined spaces).

➤ **Panic Disorders.** Sudden onset of extreme fear without reason.

➤ **Obsessive-Compulsive Disorder.** Persistent, irrational thoughts or repetitive behavior.

➤ **Post-Traumatic Stress.** Prolonged anxiety after a traumatic event.

➤ **Generalized or Free-Floating Anxiety.** Inexplicable feeling of uneasiness (affects twice as many women as men).

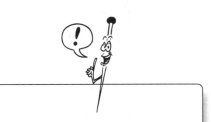

Acu-Moment

During an ordinary activity, your heart pounds and you hyperventilate, sweat, and tremble. You may think it's a heart attack, but it's a **panic disorder** that afflicts about 35 percent of Americans each year. No one is sure why these attacks occur. They typically begin between the ages of 15 and 25.

Anxiety Checklist

Anxiety affects most people from their teenage years to middle age, but others are affected at different times in their lives. Often people self-medicate with alcohol or recreational drugs to help them feel better. If you have any questions after looking over the following list, make an appointment with your health provider to discuss your feelings.

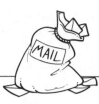

Mailbag

Joan was a 39-year-old professional who had developed free-floating anxiety, a chronic sense of uneasiness. Her family life had all the usual stresses, plus she held a demanding job. She couldn't explain it, but she did not feel comfortable or able to relax. Acupuncture treatments were given once weekly for five weeks. She began to feel better and did acupressure and Qi Gong breathing exercises at home. Now she is able to handle the challenges that her teenage children throw her way and can sleep well at night.

Symptoms of anxiety include the following:

➤ Heart palpitations

➤ Sense of impending doom

➤ Difficulty concentrating

➤ Muscle aches and chronic tension

➤ Diarrhea

➤ Hyperventilating

➤ Low sex drive

➤ Insomnia

➤ Dry mouth

➤ Chest pain

➤ Irritability

➤ Excessive sweating

➤ Under- or overeating

In school-age children, symptoms might include

➤ Fear of being away from the family.

➤ Refusal to go to school.

➤ Fear of strangers.

➤ Fear of recurring nightmares.

➤ Unnecessary worry.

Hold Down Anxiety with Oriental Medicine

Chronic uneasiness seems to be a growing concern with my patients, and fortunately they've found relief with the tools of Oriental Medicine. There are a variety of traditional oriental diagnoses that reflect the patterns of anxiety that I see in my office. Those with kidney-yin deficient anxiety, for example, have mental restlessness, often from excessive fear, guilt, shock, or overwork. A sense of anxiety, lack of willpower, insomnia, and night sweats are also characteristics of kidney-yin deficient anxiety.

Acupuncture and acupressure can bring quick relief to symptoms of anxiety. By strengthening your body with herbal medicine, exercise, and solid nutrition, you can go a long way toward leveling off anxiety. Home acupressure self-care and breathing exercises can help relieve acute anxiety episodes and give your confidence a boost.

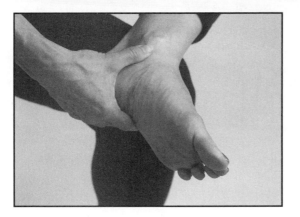

Axing anxiety.

Locate KID-6 (Shining Sea) directly below the tip of the inside anklebone. Hold this point as you breathe deeply through your nose for four counts and out through your mouth for four counts. Repeat several times until your anxiety passes.

I believe that there is comfort in knowing where to find help when you're struggling with emotional issues. Carefully consider the role you would like your acu-pro to play and discuss it to make sure your expectations are being met with the desired clarity and support. Now, let's move forward and discuss a few more conditions that require considerable support during a challenging healing process.

The Least You Need to Know

➤ Stress is common, but if left unchecked it can lead to more serious health concerns.

➤ Acu-points in the ear can ease the mind and strip away stress.

➤ Poor digestion, fatigue, and a failing memory could be due to worry. See your acu-pro for relief.

➤ Deep-breathing medical Qi Gong can lift your spirits from depression.

➤ Anxiety results from fight–or–flight reactions to no specific threat or concern.

211

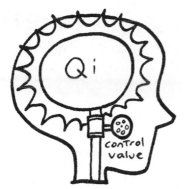

Chapter 22

Driving Your Qi: The Passing, Middle, or Breakdown Lane

In This Chapter

➤ Learn how acupuncture is helping addicts kick their habits

➤ Discover the help that's available through Oriental Medicine to people living with HIV and AIDS

➤ Lower your blood pressure by applying pressure to acu-points

➤ Find relief from chronic fatigue syndrome using acu-points and herbs

Do you have your Qi running pedal to the metal? Does your energy lurch forward like a rocketing drag racer with high blood pressure, or does your chronic fatigue engine cough and sputter as you crawl out of the starting gate? In this chapter, you'll discover the help that Oriental Medicine has been giving to all kinds of Qi drivers, including those who stay in one lane or those who weave across all three lanes because of an addition to harmful substances.

The immune-stimulating effects of acupuncture are now being used to help people with HIV/AIDS. Pull over to the nearest rest stop, and flip to the next page. There you will find the key to regulating your Qi. Happy trails!

Addiction Management: When the Party's Over

Addictions can definitely take you from flying in the fast lane to being busted in the breakdown lane. The most common substances individuals abuse—cigarettes, alcohol, and narcotics—are responsible for serious physical and health problems in our world today. Take cigarettes, for example. The nicotine in cigarettes is highly addictive. It is both a stimulant and sedative for the central nervous system. When nicotine enters your system, the almost-immediate "kick" comes from the discharge of epinephrine from the adrenal cortex. But the effects are short-lived. Depression and fatigue follow, creating a "need" to pump it up again with another puff. Under stress, hormonal corticosteroids are naturally released by your body's fight-or-flight technique, which reduces the effect of nicotine. Therefore, the more stressed you are, the more cigarettes you must smoke to achieve the same "high."

In 1998, 60 million adult Americans were cigarette smokers, and 4.1 million were between the ages of 12 and 17.

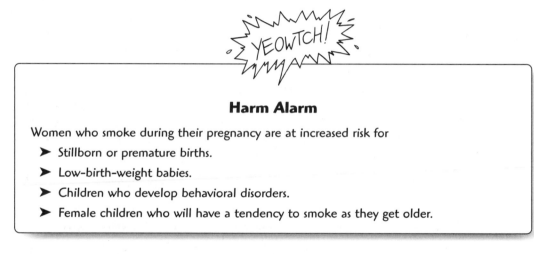

Harm Alarm

Women who smoke during their pregnancy are at increased risk for

➤ Stillborn or premature births.

➤ Low-birth-weight babies.

➤ Children who develop behavioral disorders.

➤ Female children who will have a tendency to smoke as they get older.

And then there are drugs. Drugs can be abused whether they are bought on the street corner or in the pharmacy. There is an increasing variety of drugs being abused in our country, but one of the faster-growing problems is heroin use due to higher quality and lower prices. More children in grades 8 through 12 are using heroin than ever before, some believe due to the preference for snorting and smoking rather than injecting.

In 1997 an estimated 1.5 million Americans, age 12 and older, were cocaine users. According to the National Institute of Drug Abuse, behavior associated with drug abuse such as sharing unsterilized needles is now the single largest factor in the spread of HIV infection in the United States.

The Sobering Facts on Alcoholism

The following facts come from the U.S. Department of Health and Human Services, National Institute of Alcohol Abuse and Alcoholism, and the Substance Abuse and Mental Health Services Administration:

➤ Alcohol is the most widely used drug in the U.S.

➤ Alcohol contributes to 100,000 deaths annually and is the third-leading cause of preventable death.

➤ Sixty-two percent of high school seniors report that they have been intoxicated.

➤ People who begin drinking before age 15 are four times more likely to develop alcoholism than those who begin at age 21.

➤ Current use of alcohol is highest among women ages 26–34.

➤ On average, untreated alcoholics incur general healthcare costs at least 100 percent higher than nonalcoholics.

➤ Fetal alcohol syndrome (FAS), which affects the babies of women who drink during pregnancy, is the leading cause of mental retardation in the western world.

Acupuncture and Addiction

Acupuncture has been used in private clinics to help patients in the United States deal with addictions since the early 1970s. The first hospital-based program that I'm aware of began about 17 years ago in the Bronx, New York, at Lincoln Hospital. Since then, programs have sprung up throughout this country and the world that model the protocols and successes of Lincoln Hospital's program.

Michael Smith, M.D., began and still administers the acupuncture detox program at that hospital. The program combines treatment of five-needle ear acupuncture and herbal detox tea, along with case managers to coordinate conventional health and substance abuse counseling, social services, urinalysis, and a recommended 12-step program in Narcotics and/or Alcoholics Anonymous. The ear acupuncture alters the blood and brain chemistry of dopamine receptors and other neurotransmitters. After treatment, the patients can opt for tiny, stainless steel balls taped in their ears. In between treatments, they can press on these balls to simulate the relaxation they experienced during acupuncture, which will help them through the detox. The acupuncture detox protocol is for the patients to have acupuncture treatment six days a week, whether they're trying to quit using tobacco, alcohol, heroin, or crack. During the course of the next four to six weeks, the treatments can taper off as the patients successfully detox and move on to relapse prevention.

To locate a qualified practitioner or an accredited detox clinic, contact the National Acupuncture Detoxification Association (NADA) at 1-800-765-NADA, or visit its Web site at www.acudetox.com.

Acupuncture detox is safe for pregnant women who may have difficulty being admitted into other programs. The cost is only a fraction of that for relapse conventional treatments, and the results seem quite promising.

Five needles are used for the standard detox treatment. The patient's individual health needs determine which additional ear or body acupoints will be used.

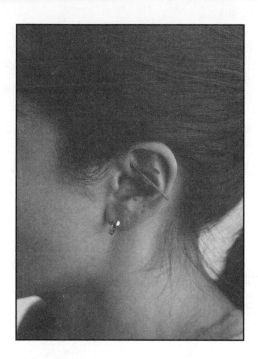

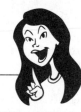

Wise Words

Acupuncture stands the test of time. A New York study of 70 people under court orders to receive acupuncture detox showed that 70 percent had clean urine samples after one year of detox. With conventional treatment, relapse in alcoholics is usually 50 percent and 80 percent in cocaine users.

HIV/AIDS: A Helping Hand for the Immune System

AIDS, or Acquired Immune Deficiency Syndrome, is a disease that reduces the body's ability to defend itself. Human immunodeficiency virus (HIV), the virus that causes AIDS, invades key immune cells called T lymphocytes and causes the entire immune system to malfunction. Once this occurs, a person living with HIV/AIDS has to stay as healthy and fit as possible because his or her system could eventually become overwhelmed with serious infections that are the leading cause of AIDS deaths.

No one knows where the virus that causes AIDS/HIV first developed, but documented cases appeared in 1981 with suspected unidentified cases in the 1970s. The virus spreads through sexual or blood-to-blood contact. It may take up to four weeks after exposure to the virus for antibodies to show up in the blood, which means that the body has recognized the invader and attempted to mount a defense against it.

Testing positive for HIV means you have contracted the virus, but not necessarily that you have developed AIDS. An AIDS diagnosis requires the presence of one or more opportunistic infections or cancers associated with HIV and AIDS. So far, only 50–60 percent of individuals who have contracted HIV have developed AIDS. The CDC reported in December 1999 that the cumulative number of AIDS cases in this country was at 688,200, with 570,425 being male, 109,311 female, and 8,461 reported as children under age 13.

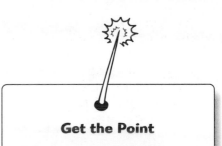

Get the Point

Help stop those cigarette cravings. A survey of 60 patients at the Midwest Acupuncture Center showed 80 percent of the two-pack-a-day smokers had a dramatic drop in smoking. Of those who smoked less, 50 percent noticed less of a change.

Oriental Medicine Manages the Immune System

I have certainly seen the benefits of treating HIV/AIDS with acupuncture and herbal medicines in my office, benefits that are reported by other practitioners who treat HIV and AIDS throughout the United States and around the world. I give each new patient an initial exam outlining the patterns of disharmony in Oriental Medical terms. It's important to learn the overall health and specific immune strength of the patient. Remember that Oriental Medicine can't promise to weaken or kill the HIV virus. Its strength is in increasing your body's immunity and overall health.

Most clinical programs see patients once per week, but more treatments may be necessary depending on the patient's health; treatments might slow down to once or twice a month over an extended period of time.

Many of the secondary infections and symptoms of HIV/AIDS can be treated with acupuncture and herbs. About 75 percent of gastrointestinal conditions such as appetite, digestion, bowel problems, and weight stabilizations, show improvement; patients also report reductions in pain, fevers, night sweats, sore throats, and sleep disorders.

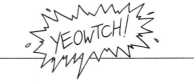

Harm Alarm

Stay safe and be aware. According to the Centers for Disease Control (CDC), roughly 200,000 Americans are unaware they are infected with HIV, the virus that causes AIDS.

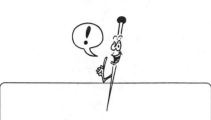

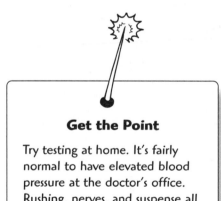

Hypertension: The Pressure's On

When the pressure is on, does your blood pressure rise? It probably does. It's normal to have blood pressure rise and fall throughout a day of changing activities and emotions. The problem comes when the force of blood pushing against your arterial walls remains consistently high, as in hypertension.

Blood pressure is measured by a sphygmomanometer. A normal reading is about 120/80; a reading of 140/90 measured at least on two office visits is officially considered high blood pressure. Hypertension rarely exhibits symptoms, so it's often called "the silent killer." Left untreated, high blood pressure can lead to serious conditions such as vision problems, heart attack, stroke, or kidney failure. If early symptoms do occur, they may include headaches, sweating, muscle cramping, palpitations, rapid pulse rate, dizziness, vision problems, or shortness of breath. Having your blood pressure checked every four to six months is an easy precaution to ensure your pressure is staying on course.

Acu-Points to Let the Steam Out

Successful treatment of high blood pressure is a balance between healthcare and self-care. I would remind you that lifestyle changes are important for long-term stabilization of hypertension. Consistent exercise, weight management, quitting or cutting back on the use of tobacco, nicotine, caffeine, and salt, and adding potassium by eating fruits and vegetables are just a few of the recommendations I normally suggest.

In Oriental Medical theory, high blood pressure is usually a combination of weakness (deficient kidney yin or yang) that gives rise to the imbalances of our blood vessels. This is one of the areas that makes the most traditional theoretical sense because your Qi is carried and circulates within your blood. Deficient kidney yin or yang are common conditions that are treated in my office with good results if consistency is applied in and out of the clinic. The channel theory of Qi is a little easier to explain in hypertension because relieving pressure in our bodies' pipes or channels is easier to envision. Your individual Oriental Medical diagnosis will determine where the imbalances lie, and your acu-pro will choose the acu-points and herbs to bring down the pressure. There are no set acu-points or Chinese herbs for hypertension, although there are commonly used points such as the ones I discuss in this chapter.

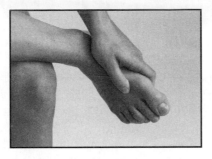

Relaxing and relieving hypertension.

Locate LIV-3 (Great Pouring), which is in the webbing between the first large toe and the second. Using the opposite side's thumb, press firmly into the sorest spot for one to two minutes. Breathe deeply, repeating two to four times per session. Other points to help hypertension include KD-3 (see Chapter 23, "Balancing Your Qi—Too Much Here, Not Enough There") and GB-20 (see Chapter 7, "Pain From the Neck Up").

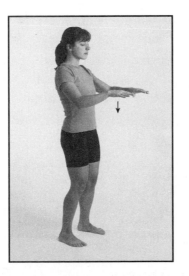

Relaxing and relieving hypertension.

Stand with your feet at about shoulder width, knees slightly bent, and eyes closed. Imagine a string is holding you up, running from the top of your head through your body to the floor. Turn your palms up and gently lift them as you breathe deeply in through your nose. When your palms reach the center of your chest, turn them over,

219

breathe out slowly through your mouth, and pretend you are pushing down on a tabletop that lowers to the floor with your gentle pressure. Feel the tingling and warmth in your palms. Allow your mind and muscles to let go as you repeat this technique three to five times daily to achieve relaxation and to help keep the pressure off.

Chronic Fatigue Syndrome ... or Just Plain Tired

An item on almost every patient's wish list is more energy. As we cut back on sleep and add more activities, such as our children's sports, to an already crowded week, guess what? We run out of gas. I always ask if the amount of fatigue you feel is realistic given what you've just put yourself through. When you weigh it all out, does it make sense? If it doesn't, then you could be looking at a potential medical condition.

Chronic fatigue immune dysfunction syndrome (CFIDS) first came to the public's attention in the mid-1980s. It primarily strikes young people between the ages of 25 and 40, with women under 45 accounting for 80 percent of the cases. CFIDS is characterized by overwhelming fatigue and other flulike symptoms. It is not contagious and does not result from overexertion. Symptoms can be sudden and debilitating, but are not fatal. There is no known cause. Theories of a connection between CFIDS and Epstein-Barr virus (which causes mononucleosis) are apparently unfounded.

Chronic Fatigue Checklist

The condition is clinically evaluated for symptoms that have persisted or reoccurred during six or more consecutive months and were not present before your fatigue. Recurrence of four or more of the following symptoms suggest you may have CFIDS:

➤ Unexplained persistent or relapsing fatigue, not brought on by exertion or alleviated by rest

➤ Substantial impairment of short-term memory or concentration

➤ Sore throat

➤ Tender lymph nodes

➤ Muscle pain

➤ Multijoint pain, swelling, or redness

➤ Nonrefreshing sleep

➤ Headaches that you've never had before

➤ Fatigue for more than 24 hours after exercise

Acu-Points to Relieve the Fatigue

Oriental Medicine is particularly well suited to look at your chronic fatigue. Work with your acu-pro to figure out a treatment strategy that realistically meets your expectations and goals. I'm a provider for the Fibromyalgia/CFIDS Network, which connects members with qualified practitioners who understand and frequently treat those conditions.

Your CFIDS symptoms may be similar to others with the same diagnosis, but your overall health will determine the Oriental Medical pattern that needs attention and the treatment plan that will be customized for you. Your acu-pro, in considering the patterns below, also includes the CFIDS symptoms listed earlier in this chapter. Common CFIDS patterns include

➤ **Lung Qi deficiency.** Easily catch colds, low voice, pale complexion, spontaneous sweating, and pale tongue.

➤ **Spleen yang deficiency.** Fatigue, muscular weakness, poor appetite, cold limbs, loose bowels, and slight abdominal ache.

➤ **Heart blood deficiency.** Tiredness that is worse at midday, palpitation, poor memory, insomnia, dizziness, and dream-disturbed sleep.

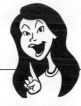

Wise Words

The Fibromyalgia/CFIDS Network provides members with the latest recommended treatments and provider lists for this condition. Acupuncture is frequently mentioned as a viable treatment option. Check Appendix D, "State and National Organizations," for their contact information.

➤ **Lung yin deficiency.** Dry throat, dry cough, exhausting breathlessness, hoarse voice, afternoon feeling of overheating, sweating in palms, feet, and center of chest, night sweats, and flushed face.

The conditions we've just discussed take consistent effort and follow-through to achieve desirable results. I believe that Oriental Medicine can make a significant contribution to your health, and would also urge you to incorporate an entire health team to bring the best possible care during the course of your treatments. But don't fall asleep on me now because we talk about insomnia, weight loss, and other tricky conditions in the next chapter!

The Least You Need to Know

➤ Acupuncture detox clinics effectively treat drug, alcohol, and tobacco addictions.

➤ HIV/AIDS patients believe acupuncture and herbs are important parts of their healthcare.

➤ Bring down high blood pressure, the silent killer, with acu-point therapy.

➤ Your CFIDS symptoms can improve greatly and be well maintained with Oriental Medicine.

Chapter 23

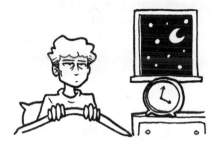

Balancing Your Qi—Too Much Here, Not Enough There

In This Chapter

➤ Sleep soundly with Oriental Medicine

➤ Acu-points rescue you from the cold of Raynaud's Phenomenon

➤ Tone down tinnitus with herbs and acu-points

➤ Acu-points and exercise: your tag team to wrestle weight loss

---

Keeping your life in balance can be quite a challenge in the twenty-first century. I often explain to patients that their healing progress may be more enjoyable if they check into a spa for a month or two. Instead, most of us are doing our best to heal our bodies and minds in the process of living. Our jobs, kids, pets, car problems, noisy neighbors, unsympathetic supervisors, and mortgages make up the balance of the imbalances we call our normal lives. The challenge: to keep up the healing while we continue the dealing.

This chapter deals with the imbalances that result from not getting enough sleep, gaining too much weight, developing poor blood circulation, and having too much noise in your ears. Your life is still yours to figure out, but perhaps it's comforting to know that I've found some ways to help with these conditions to lighten your load a bit. You can start out this chapter very balanced. Place both feet squarely on the floor, grasp the book with a relaxed yet firm hold (even with the middle of your torso), and get ready to start turning pages. See you at the other end.

Insomnia: Cruisin' for a Snoozin'

There's nothing more refreshing than to greet the day after a good night's sleep. It's equally frustrating to be part of the estimated one-third of Americans (twice as many women than men) that suffer from some form of insomnia. Seniors make up about 50 percent of all those who suffer from sleep disorders, but I'm seeing a growing number of adolescents and adults who complain of poor sleep or wake up feeling unrefreshed.

Most of us have experienced difficulty falling or staying asleep due to a late meal, excitement, or worry. Other potential causes of insomnia include hypoglycemia, pain, breathing problems, caffeine, jet lag, and some medications. Chronic insomnia can make your days seem like months and any activity you undertake feels like an uphill battle.

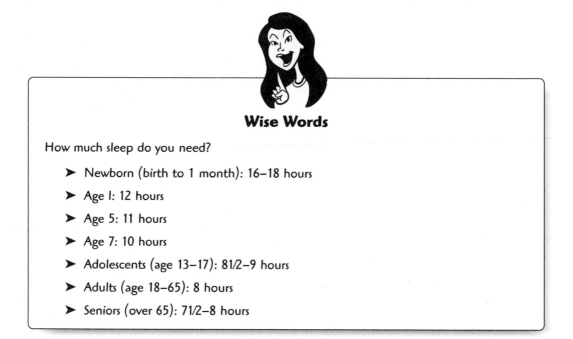

Wise Words

How much sleep do you need?

➤ Newborn (birth to 1 month): 16–18 hours

➤ Age 1: 12 hours

➤ Age 5: 11 hours

➤ Age 7: 10 hours

➤ Adolescents (age 13–17): 81/2–9 hours

➤ Adults (age 18–65): 8 hours

➤ Seniors (over 65): 71/2–8 hours

Normal sleep is composed of REM (rapid eye movement) sleep and NREM (nonrapid eye movement) sleep. During REM sleep, we dream, lose muscle tone, and have irregular heartbeat and breathing. During NREM sleep, we do not dream, maintain muscle tone, and have regular heartbeat and breathing. During a normal night's sleep, you will cycle through both kinds of sleep. About 30 minutes after falling asleep, you enter NREM; an hour later you go to REM sleep. The deepest and most restful sleep occurs during NREM, when your body is the least active.

There are about 80 different sleep disorders affecting approximately 70 million Americans, including

➤ **Psychological insomnia.** Caused by mental and emotional stress.

➤ **Sleep apnea.** Intense snoring caused by blocked breathing passages that disrupts sleep; as a result, patients wake up as many as 200 times per night.

➤ **Restless leg syndrome.** Discomfort in calves and thighs, resulting in frequent leg movements and jerking that disturb sleep.

➤ **Narcolepsy.** Sudden, daytime attacks of severe sleepiness.

Acu-Points to Soothe You to Sleep

I see this as a growing concern with my patients. Poor sleep can be a part of many other conditions such as anxiety, depression, stress, or hormonal imbalances. With an increased workload at home and at work, many of my patients are choosing to cut back on sleep to get more done during the day. The resulting imbalance can be corrected by using acu-points and a few easy-to-follow sleep tips.

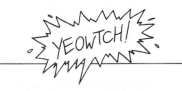

Harm Alarm

Watch your intake of alcohol and narcotics. Alcohol can help you relax and fall asleep, but it often causes you to wake up in the middle of the night. Fifty percent of people who regularly take sleeping pills worsen their insomnia. Chronic sleeping pill users are 50 percent more likely to die in automobile accidents than nonusers.

Oriental Medicine takes a look at your overall health patterns and factors them into your sleep disorder. We first separate the sleep problems: difficulty falling asleep (deficient blood condition), staying asleep (deficient yin condition), or both (deficient blood and yin). Sleep position is examined as well.

If you can't sleep on your back, then we suspect excess condition of lungs or heart; if you can only sleep on your back with outstretched arms, excess heat; sleeping on your stomach would indicate a deficiency, possibly of the stomach; on your side points to deficient Qi or blood. Snoring—which affects 25 percent of men and 15 percent of women—is characterized by excess phlegm of the stomach channel. For all of these conditions, I've found that acu-points and/or Chinese herbal medicine bring great relief.

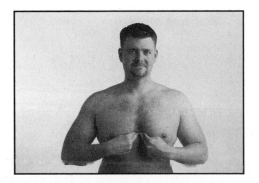

Inducing sleep.

225

Stabilize your hands by laying them on your chest, gently at first, pressing into CV-17 located in the middle of the sternum between the nipples. Press gently, adjusting the pressure to your comfort. This acu-point clears the heart, calms the mind, and promotes sleep.

Inducing sleep.

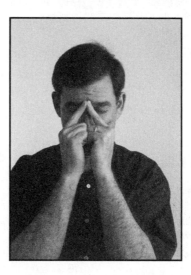

Locate Yintang (Seal Hall) in between your eyebrows. Use your index fingers to gently press the point for 30 seconds while closing your eyes and breathing deeply. Repeat three to five times. Your free hand can cradle your elbow to keep your pressing arm relaxed if you choose to press with only one finger. This acu-point releases heat and wind and is used to calm your mind. Additional acu-points to aid insomnia include CU-4, PC-6, and SP-6 (see Chapter 16, "Birthing Baby"), and HT-7 and LIV-3 (see Chapter 18, "Female Frustrations").

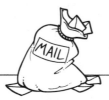

Mailbag

Kathy complained of poor sleep due to restless leg syndrome. Each night her legs would feel tighter as the night progressed, and she found herself stretching, rolling over, and waking many times. Her anxiety at bedtime was also growing. We began acupuncture treatments, which helped relax her muscles and mind. Within two weeks, she noticed a great change in her sleep pattern. At the end of six weeks, she was sleeping through the night. She now uses stretching excercises and acupressure as her self-care and has not counted sheep for months.

Better Sleep Checklist

The acupressure points described for insomnia ought to help you get some *z's*. But if you need more help, here are a few more tips:

➤ Go to bed when you're tired, not before.

➤ Avoid napping during the day.

➤ Use your bedroom for sleeping or romance; cut out the TV, eating, or working.

➤ Get up at the same time every day, even on weekends, to help set and maintain your body clock.

➤ Exercise regularly during the day, but do not take part in vigorous exercise three hours or less before bedtime.

➤ Avoid caffeine, alcohol, and nicotine in the evening hours.

➤ Get out of bed if you can't sleep; move around or do something else until you are sleepy, and then return to bed.

➤ Learn relaxation techniques to put worry and stress on the nightstand until morning comes.

Raynaud's Phenomenon: When the Cold Gets Old

The next time you reach into your refrigerator, imagine seeing your fingers turn white, and then blue as a sudden wave of extreme cold overtakes your hand. If you have *Raynaud's Phenomenon,* you don't have to imagine this condition because you live with it. Raynaud's affects mostly women between the ages of 15 and 50. Researchers believe that those afflicted with this condition have blood vessels that overreact to cold, but they do not understand why this occurs. Cold temperatures are more likely to attack when you are physically or emotionally stressed. For some, stress alone can cause the cold.

Primary Raynaud's usually affects both hands and both feet and is not connected to another disorder. Secondary Raynaud's symptoms are part of other conditions or medications such as scleroderma, a thickening of the skin; systemic lupus, chronic inflammation of the skin; rheumatoid arthritis, chronic inflammation and swelling of tissue in the joints; nerve problems or the side effects of heart, blood, or migraine medications.

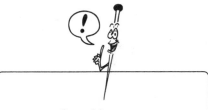

Acu-Moment

Raynaud's Phenomenon is a disorder of the small blood vessels that feed the skin. During an attack, arteries briefly contract, causing skin to turn white, then blue. Your skin turns red as arteries relax and let the blood and oxygen flow again. Hands and feet are the most common areas affected, but the nose and ears are also possible targets.

227

Remedies for the Extremities: The Oriental Medical Viewpoint

Raynaud's Phenomenon can be one of the most frustrating conditions that someone has to deal with. The sudden overwhelming cold a person feels in the extremities occurs year-round with any exposure to cold temperatures. I, of course, see the patients who do not respond satisfactorily to medications or to prevention techniques like wearing scarves, mittens, warm socks, and boots.

Fortunately, Oriental Medicine has a few techniques to help keep the flow aglow. After the initial visit to determine overall health and find the oriental pattern of imbalance, I often use combinations of acupuncture and Chinese herbs, along with home- and self-care measures like acupressure, Tai Chi, and biomagnets. These treatments will stimulate your body's ability to maintain normal levels of circulation regardless of the temperature. A qualified herbalist will put together a custom prescription based on your complete health. Chinese herbs that I often use include millettia root and vine (Ji Zue Teng), Szechuan lounge root (Chuan Xiong), dried ginger root (Gan Jiang), cinnamon inner bark (Rou Gui), milk vetch root (Huang Qi), and vine of Solomon's seal (Ye Jiao Teng). Therapeutic doses of herbs need to be combined and balanced in a formula by your herbalist to ensure safety and best results.

Dealing with Raynaud's Phenomenon.

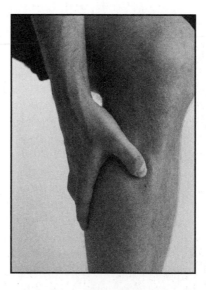

Locate ST-36 (Three Measures on the Leg), which is four-finger width below the kneecap and one-finger width to the outside. Use index and middle fingers or thumbs, firmly pressing for one to two minutes. Breathe deep, gentle breaths, and rub the point after pressing.

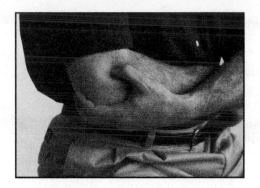

Dealing with Raynaud's Phenomenon.

Locate LI-11 (Crooked Pool); with the arm bent at the elbow, the acu-point is on the outside of the elbow, halfway between the elbow crease and bone that sticks out. Press for one to two minutes, breathing deeply. This acu-point helps increase circulation in the arm and hand.

Tinnitus: The Ring You Can't Answer

Ringing, buzzing, hissing, chirping, and whistling ... will it ever stop? For an estimated 50 million Americans with tinnitus, commonly called "ringing in the ears," it doesn't. I have lectured to hospital-based tinnitus support groups and heard the word about this incredibly annoying and aggravating condition. The ear noises can be intermittent or continuous, and the loudness also varies. Background noises of daily life often drown out the ringing or buzzing during the day. The worst time seems to be when you're trying to fall asleep in a quiet room. The noises can be so distracting that they interfere with your concentration, work, relationships, and sleeping patterns. For many, the personal distress creates anxiety about going to bed at night. Tinnitus is often associated with hearing loss, but it does not cause the loss, nor does hearing loss cause tinnitus. The cause of tinnitus is obscure.

Turn On Your Acu-Points, Shut Off the Ringer

Using the tools and techniques of Oriental Medicine, you and your acu-pro can effectively manage tinnitus so that you will hardly notice the noise inside your head. While I've not been successful in every case, the number of people who have been helped is growing.

The two most common oriental diagnoses of tinnitus that I see are rising liver and gallbladder fire, and kidney deficiency. Rising liver and gallbladder fire is characterized by sudden onset of a loud noise, emotional stress, headache, irritability, a bitter taste in the mouth, constipation, dizziness, reddish face, and thirst. Deficient kidney tinnitus comes on gradually with low, intermittent sounds, poor memory, blurred vision, sore back and knees, and reduced sexual desire or performance.

I've had patients express satisfaction after being treated for both of these conditions. Some courses of treatment are longer, especially with the deficient kidney, because you're building up an internal weakness that has been developed over the years.

In this case acupuncture, acupressure, and herbs are used to achieve two treatment goals. First, they work to bring down the rising Qi fire that in Oriental Medical theory is responsible for the noises. Second, and not to be forgotten, is the desire to strengthen and balance your body's own overall health so that your natural checks and balances will occur. Your patience and persistence will grow as your condition improves, and ringing, chirping, and all the other ear noises will be sounds of the past.

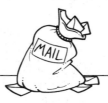

Mailbag

Sally was 68, widowed, and retired. She was looking forward to a peaceful life of helping her daughter with the new grandchildren and volunteering in her community. She'd had tinnitus for almost 20 years, but the ringing had been getting louder and more bothersome, causing her great distress. We began a series of acupuncture treatments, two times weekly for one month. She began to steadily experience less ringing and better sleep. She used herbal medicine, acupressure, and biomagnets at home; acupuncture treatments were cut back to once a week. Within two and a half months, the ringing was hardly noticeable.

Managing tinnitus.

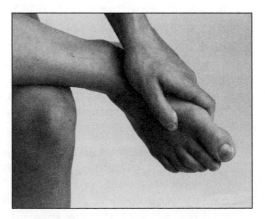

Locate LIV-3 (Great Pouring) in the webbing between the first and second toes. Using the opposite side's thumb, press firmly into the sorest spot for one to two minutes. Breathe deeply, repeating two to four times per session. These acu-points are used for treating tinnitus caused by rising liver and gallbladder fire. Other relevant acu-points include KD-1 (see Chapter 17, "The Disappointment Down Under") and LI-4 (see Chapter 16).

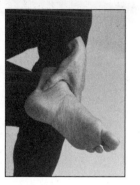

Managing tinnitus.

Locate KD-3 (Great Creek) directly behind the inside anklebone in the middle of the Achilles tendon. Press firmly while breathing deeply for one to two minutes. Repeat three to five times each session. This point is used to strengthen kidney energy. Other acu-points for kidney-deficient tinnitus include CV-4 and SP-6 (see Chapter 16).

Weight Management: Motorize Your Metabolism

We close this chapter on imbalances with perhaps our country's greatest health challenge: weight management. We look in a mirror, step on a scale, or put on our bathing suit, and what runs through our minds? Too fat! Too thin! Body imaging is a large-scale issue in this country and goes well beyond the scope of this chapter.

Weight management is at a crisis level in our country. It is estimated by the U.S. Centers for Disease Control and Prevention that one-third of Americans are 20 percent or more overweight, which qualifies them as being obese. National surveys show that 25–50 percent of adults are on diets and spend about $30 billion each year on them. Unfortunately, a lot of that money goes to waste without the proper lifestyle changes. Two-thirds of those who lose weight will gain it back during the next three to five years. The average human body has 30–40 billion fat cells, which are genetically geared for helping you store unused calories. It's simple: Use those calories, or they go into storage … visible storage!

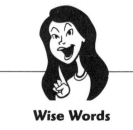

Wise Words

A woman's body is designed to store fat for pregnancy and nursing during famine. Fat can make up to 25 percent of a healthy woman's body weight and 17 percent of a man's.

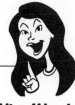

Wise Words

Obesity is defined as being 20 percent over normal body weight for your age, sex, and height. Common causes of obesity include

➤ Poor diet and eating habits.

➤ Lack of consistent vigorous exercise.

➤ Glandular malfunction.

➤ Diabetes.

➤ Hypoglycemia.

➤ Emotional stress.

➤ Boredom.

Acu-Points for Better Digestion and Food Cravings

I always make it clear to patients that while acupuncture can be good for improving your metabolism, it is no substitution for proper nutrition and exercise. Let's make that clear up front.

The responsible way to use acu-points is to jump-start your digestion if it's sluggish, and then back off the treatments once you've created a lifestyle that leads you to your ideal weight. First off, I recommend throwing away the scale, ignoring clothing sizes, and going by your energy level, endurance, and how your clothes fit. Scales are a poor measure of success and, in my opinion, lead to premature disappointment and frustration.

Improving digestion.

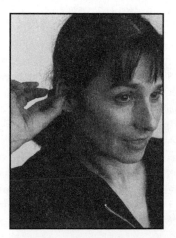

Locate the stomach point on your ear, which is in the middle of the ear on the horizontal raised ridge called the crus of the helix. Squeeze the point with your finger on the point and your thumb behind for support. You may also use your fingernail, as shown in the previous figure, for greater stimulation, but be careful not to press too hard and break the skin. Squeeze the point to curb your appetite or help you resist a food craving. Squeeze for one to two minutes, breathing deeply. Repeat three to five times per session.

The New Truth About Exercise

I can tell the times I've been into exercising by the number of machines, bars, racks, and widgets that are collecting dust in my basement. All good intentions, all good money, all good things come to an end. I never found what I liked until my wife and I began mountain biking and spinning last year. We enjoy it, and we're able to do it together and make it a part of our lives. We're not perfect, but we feel a lot better. You may not lose as much weight, but you'll replace fat with muscle, and the way your clothes fit will reflect your progress.

It makes sense to get the numbers working in your favor. *The New England Journal of Medicine* studied 34 formerly obese women who lost an average of 25 pounds. Moderate to sedentary women in one year gained back from 14 to 20 pounds. They also found a surprising exercise level necessary to loose weight, long term. The women who kept the weight off averaged 80 minutes per day of moderate activity, such as brisk walking, or 35 minutes per day of vigorous activity, such as aerobics or fast cycling.

Oriental Medical philosophy has long been a proponent for healthy eating, exercise, and calming and centering the mind. The conditions we've just covered can all be frustrating and challenging, so bring in the help as early as you can and take back control of your health. We're getting ready to begin the last part of the book, "The Home Stretch." Keep on reading to find the answers to the important questions you may have on how to get started. See you there.

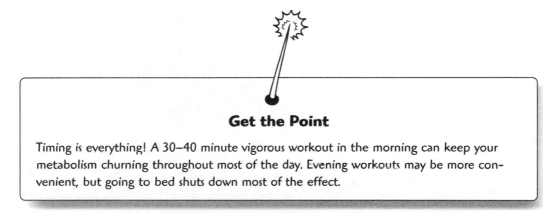

Get the Point

Timing is everything! A 30–40 minute vigorous workout in the morning can keep your metabolism churning throughout most of the day. Evening workouts may be more convenient, but going to bed shuts down most of the effect.

233

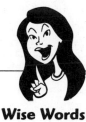

> ### Wise Words
>
> Frowns can tip the scales against you. The September 1998 issue of *Annals of Behavior Medicine* found that those who were unhappy with their bodies had the least success losing weight.

> ## The Least You Need to Know
>
> ➤ There are about 80 different sleep disorders, affecting approximately 70 million Americans.
>
> ➤ Acupuncture and acupressure can effectively treat many types of sleep problems.
>
> ➤ Oriental Medicine, including acupressure, brings much-needed circulation to sufferers of Raynaud's Phenomenon.
>
> ➤ Acu-points can curb food cravings and power your metabolism for better weight management.
>
> ➤ Eighty minutes of moderate exercise or 35 minutes of vigorous exercise daily are needed to keep the weight off.

Part 5

The Home Stretch

Now that you've either read the book or skipped around to the chapters that directly concern you, it's time to find your own personal acu-pro. This part of the book helps you understand the clues to the natural healing process, how to choose your healing crew, and what your job as the team captain might be. I'm glad your interest is peaked, and you've read this far. For a quality experience, go the distance—just a bit further. You will receive 100 percent back on this investment to your health and peace of mind. So turn the pages of this book, and I'll see you at the finish line.

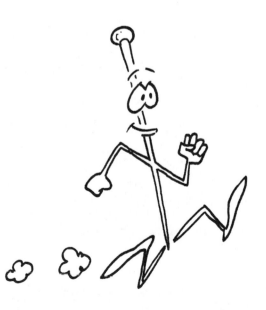

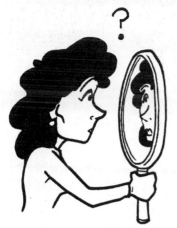

Chapter 24

Expectations—
Am I Better Yet?

In This Chapter

➤ Learn how your body heals

➤ Discover how acu-points speed up the healing process

➤ Find out how time and patience add up to better health

➤ How to make sure your acupuncture is working

Knowing what's in store for you is an important part in choosing your options for healthcare. Your body has a unique ability to continuously heal, but when something impairs this ability, symptoms develop into conditions that may require treatment. Time and patience may be difficult to muster up, given the frustrations of illness.

This chapter covers the realistic view you'll need to have in order to heal naturally. You'll want to learn how to evaluate your progress and whether it's worth your time and money. Let's get started.

The Natural Healing Process

In today's world of instant coffee, drive-thru windows, and one-hour photo development, it's easy to become impatient with the healing time needed for most conditions. Our bodies are amazingly complex systems, containing intricate, simultaneous, multi-tasking cell growth; janitorial services; repair and maintenance divisions; and a defense department to fend off dangerous invaders. Yet, why can't a cold go away faster?

After World War II, we discovered a group of medications called antibiotics that would kill disease-causing bacteria. These medications saved lives then and still do today. The challenge for us is that the magic-bullet solution to disease has some downsides—namely, antibiotic-resistant bacteria and the side effects these medications may have.

Patients I see are conflicted about what to do for their own health and healing. They want the instantaneous effect of a drug, but they want it in a natural way. Oriental Medicine often relieves symptoms quickly, but the greatest strength of this medical system is that it can help to heal the underlying conditions that led to your illness or injury. That part often takes time. Treatments are always geared to relieving the symptoms that motivated you to make the appointment, while strengthening the deficiencies or removing the excesses that block your path to continued good health.

How Acu-Points Help

Whether you're doing acupuncture, acupressure, herbal or nutritional therapy, or medical Qi Gong exercises, the idea is to jump-start your system and point it in the right direction for your optimal health. Think of acu-points as the retro-rockets on a

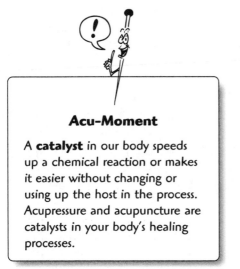

Acu-Moment

A **catalyst** in our body speeds up a chemical reaction or makes it easier without changing or using up the host in the process. Acupressure and acupuncture are catalysts in your body's healing processes.

spaceship. When you get off course, a few blasts from the rockets put you back on track. If all goes well, you'll stay that way, but if meteors, planetary gravity, or space junk interfere with your flight, activate your acu-points … I mean rockets … to help you regain your balance. I believe this to be an accurate analogy to using acu-points to achieve and maintain health. Put in more "scientific" terms, applying pressure to acu-points acts as a *catalyst* for other bodily processes.

Another story I tell patients is this. Let's say that in order to get well, you will need to jump over a 50-foot wall. This is a daunting task to take on by yourself. Using acu-points, however, lowers the wall to 10 feet. You still have to use effort to get over, only now it's possible with the helping hand of Oriental Medicine.

Limitations: How Far Can You Go?

Well, you've had acupuncture; now you can jump over tall buildings and never have to worry about your health again. Not likely! Using Oriental Medicine to assist your body's healing has its limitations. I am often asked, "How many times will I need to get treated for my back?" Unfortunately, at first, there are no easy or quick answers to that question.

After a thorough initial visit and a review of past medical diagnosis, however, I should be able to give a realistic answer. The short answer is that an acute injury without structural damage (herniated disks or fractures) responds quickly, within one to three treatments. Chronic conditions, either musculoskeletal or internal (such as asthma), can have a significant relief of symptoms within one to five visits, but may take longer to work on the underlying health concerns that keep you from feeling well all the time. A typical course of treatments for chronic conditions is 6–12 visits. Whether you are seen once or twice a week usually depends on the severity of your symptoms and the degree of disruption of everyday activities. Acu-points are marvelous tools that assist the body's healing in numerous ways, but we cannot make disks go back into the spinal column or tumors go away by themselves.

Time and Patience: Hard Medicine to Swallow

When patients come to my office, I can guess they've just about had it by the time they push open the front door. I'm like that, too, when I'm not feeling well. I have to ask you to give me the two things you're short on: time and patience. Acute injuries or sickness that can often be alleviated quickly are not taken care of quickly enough. Oriental Medicine looks at the aftermath of an acute malady. When the symptoms are gone or much diminished, what damage has been done, or what imbalance exists that will be the foundation for future illnesses? Left untreated, you will join the American Walking Wounded Club—not really sick, but not really well. Sick and tired of being sick and tired!

Pick your acu-pro's brain and ask that he or she explain your patterns to you. Knowing this information can help you understand and focus on a new level of health. It's amazing the enjoyment you can have in life when you truly feel a sense of well-being. This process will still take time and patience, but I believe you'll be rewarded in the end.

How to Tell If You're Better: Did It Work?

When I sit down with patients for our initial visit, I ask them for their wish list. We go through all the diagnostic procedures outlined in Chapter 2, "What to Expect on Your First Visit—Does It Hurt?" and then I go back to that wish list. We take the last few minutes of the visit to discuss the big picture of their health and any thoughts on how much Oriental Medicine can assist them. Next I ask them about their expectations: How fast do you expect to get well? I want to make sure their expectations match the reality of their conditions. We set appropriate goals—short-, medium-, and long-term—and begin designing a comprehensive treatment plan to get them there.

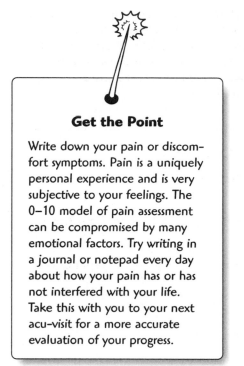

Get the Point

Write down your pain or discomfort symptoms. Pain is a uniquely personal experience and is very subjective to your feelings. The 0–10 model of pain assessment can be compromised by many emotional factors. Try writing in a journal or notepad every day about how your pain has or has not interfered with your life. Take this with you to your next acu-visit for a more accurate evaluation of your progress.

At the beginning of each visit, we discuss your progress to make sure you're on course to feeling well. In most cases, I give myself about six to eight visits to determine if Oriental Medicine is the right approach for your condition. Depending on the complaints, I don't always expect you to be completely better by then, but I acknowledge that for both of us to continue other treatments, we both must recognize that we've made verifiable progress.

Fortunately, the notes from our initial visit serve as a reminder of your former condition. We can review your pain-scale reading, range of motion, symptoms, and changes in tongue, pulse, and skin since the treatment began. As we check things off on your wish list, we often have less and less to talk about regarding your health. That's a good thing. Treatment appointments are spaced out with you doing more self-care. As your condition improves, you'll see that your investment of time and energy into your lifestyle does make a difference.

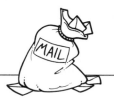

Mailbag

Frank was 43 years old and complained of not being able to do his work or have fun because of his chronic back pain and sciatica. Frank had been diagnosed with herniated disks at L-3 through S-1 of his low back, with burning sciatica extending from his left buttock down the back of his legs to his toes. Pain began to hit him by two or three o'clock in the afternoon as he worked on his feet. The pain even prevented him from going fishing, which was his favorite way to unwind. We began acupuncture treatments twice a week for about three weeks. He felt reduced levels of pain and greater endurance at work. We cut treatments back to once per week, then every other week, and finally once per month. Acupuncture can't cure his herniated disks, but it's the best pain management tool he's used. He's been fishing every weekend since the treatment began.

In today's instant Internet era it's been more challenging for me to discuss the natural process of healing when my patients can order overnight products from around the world. We're used to getting what we want, when we want it. Our bodies do have a say in all this. They ultimately dictate the progress we make in healing. Having a good team with you on this journey is essential in my book. Hey, this is my book! Anyway, let's examine the components of a healing team.

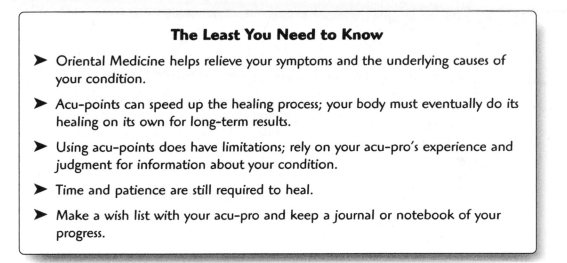

The Least You Need to Know

➤ Oriental Medicine helps relieve your symptoms and the underlying causes of your condition.

➤ Acu-points can speed up the healing process; your body must eventually do its healing on its own for long-term results.

➤ Using acu-points does have limitations; rely on your acu-pro's experience and judgment for information about your condition.

➤ Time and patience are still required to heal.

➤ Make a wish list with your acu-pro and keep a journal or notebook of your progress.

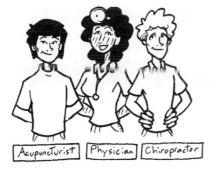

Chapter 25

Acupuncturist | Physician | Chiropractor

Building a Winning Team

> ## In This Chapter
>
> ➤ Learn how to choose the acu-pro who's right for you
>
> ➤ Your doctor may or may not be interested in Oriental Medicine; find out how to start the conversation
>
> ➤ Discover why your acu-pro doesn't go it alone
>
> ➤ Learn to lean on a shoulder of solid support

It's action time. You are one phone call away from beginning your journey to better health, but who are you going to call? This chapter gets down to finding the best acu-pro for you. We'll also talk about telling your doctor about your big move to Oriental Medicine; it may not be as scary as you think. When do you need the assistance of someone besides your acu-pro? We'll take a look.

Finally, we cover the importance of recruiting and including your family, friends, and possibly a support group to your healing team. The starting gun has fired; read on, and you're off to better health!

Choosing Your Acu-Pro: A Needle in a Haystack

How would you find the best restaurant, barber, or car mechanic in town? I think most of us would ask a good friend. Finding out if a trusted friend, one who you know and respect, has been to or heard of a qualified acu-pro in your area is still the best and most reliable way to locate acu-help.

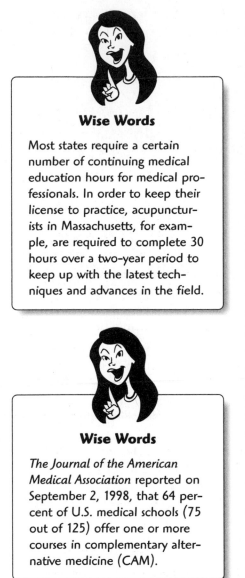

Wise Words

Most states require a certain number of continuing medical education hours for medical professionals. In order to keep their license to practice, acupuncturists in Massachusetts, for example, are required to complete 30 hours over a two-year period to keep up with the latest techniques and advances in the field.

Wise Words

The Journal of the American Medical Association reported on September 2, 1998, that 64 percent of U.S. medical schools (75 out of 125) offer one or more courses in complementary alternative medicine (CAM).

Once you start opening the door to this line of communication, you may be surprised at the number of acquaintances or coworkers who have already chosen Oriental Medicine as a part of their healthcare. If that doesn't work, I've provided you with a list of national organizations and schools in Appendixes D, "State and National Organizations," and E, "Acupuncture Schools." Graduates and members have to have a minimum level of credentials and continuing education certificates to belong, ensuring you a strong foundation and competency.

I would also call the local chamber of commerce or Rotary Club. Find out if the professional you've found is actively supporting your community. Last, I would look at advertising, but keep in mind that anyone can plop down money to buy an ad. Check out the practitioner with the schools and organizations listed.

Your next step is to make the phone call and ask if the acu-pro has experience in your particular condition. Follow your instincts. Are you reassured by his or her voice and manner? Do you feel confident about the acu-pro after your phone call? Going to your first appointment will often help you decide for sure. Then, once you've found an acu-pro you're comfortable with, enjoy the process of healing that a good practitioner can provide.

Informing Your Physician: What's Up, Doc?

I was lecturing as part of grand rounds at an area hospital when a patient mentioned that he had been seeing an acupuncturist during his cancer treatments. He went on to say that when he told his doctor during an office visit how helpful the acupuncturist had been, he got no reply. He said his doctor acted like he didn't even hear him and would not look at him again until he stopped referring to the experience he had with acupuncture. Unfortunately, this patient's experience is not an uncommon one.

According to a survey reported in the November 1998 *Journal of the American Medical Association,* less than 40 percent of alternative therapies were disclosed to medical doctors. Experiences like the one I witnessed are not new, but I believe they will be less common in the near future. There is a concerted effort being made by practitioners—both conventional and complementary—to learn more about each other's medical practices and the possibilities that exist for improving patient care through combined efforts.

A national survey performed by Landmark, a California-based insurance company, showed that 74 percent of respondents want to use alternative care along with their conventional medical care. Clearly, the shift is going toward communication and some form of integration. I believe it's essential that you give your doctor a written list of all the healthcare practitioners that you see, and any vitamins or herbs that you are taking. Why not mention your interest and interaction in Oriental Medicine to your doctor? Have your acu-pro make a phone call or send a note that he or she is seeing you as a patient. Share this book, or a recent magazine article to start off the conversation with your medical doctor. Who knows … you may find he's been looking at the same books!

Do You Need More Help?

I have a line on my new patient intake form where I ask who your primary care provider is. I also like to know the other health professionals that you are seeing so that I am sure proper attention is being paid to your condition. There are many conditions, including anxiety, depression, cancer, and AIDS, that require intense coordination between Orien-tal Medical practitioners and other healthcare providers.

In addition, there are also aspects to some cases that go beyond the scope of my training and licensure. For that, I refer to a network of trusted colleagues in my area. This list includes medical doctors (both primary and specialists), psychiatrists, social workers, chiropractors, *homeopaths,* massage therapists, and osteopaths. These professionals add a greater dimension to the healing the patient receives. I get permission from the patient so that we can all talk together and figure out a more dynamic way to assist you in feeling better.

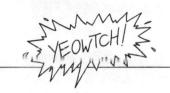

Harm Alarm

Be aware that herbs are medicines, and have the potential to interfere with any medications you're taking. Although very little research has been done to study the interaction between Chinese herbs and pharmaceutical medications, we do know, for instance, that some herbs react with antiseizure medications. Inform your herbalist and physician about what you are taking to make sure it's safe.

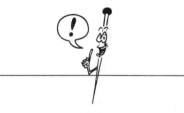

Acu-Moment

Homeopathy is a complete system of healing discovered about 200 years ago by a German physician, Dr. Samuel Hahne-mann. The remedies are all natural and prepared by diluting and shaking them to enhance their strength. They have no harmful side effects and are not addictive.

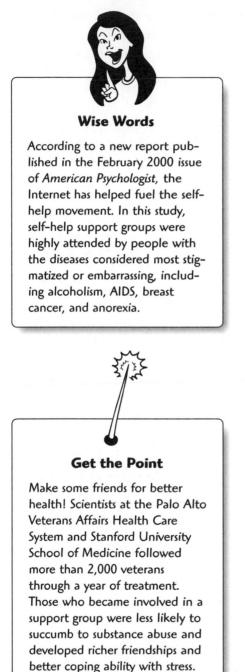

I will also let patients know when I feel I'm unable to help them, and assist them by referring to another provider if they wish. Despite my best efforts, I'm not able to satisfy every patient's needs. A talented group of colleagues waiting in the wings is the best next step to continuing your journey to wellness.

Getting the Support You Need: A Family Affair

Along with professional support, I like to know the quality of personal support you've got at home. In a serious illness, having someone to help shop, clean, and care for you is essential in conserving energy. Also, there's just something about being loved and cared for by your family and friends. I also use family in the extended sense, meaning caring neighbors, friends, or relatives that can help you out in a pinch or give you quality listening time when you need it. I've found that patients who have to go it alone have a more difficult time keeping it together during stressful or painful situations. Some of my exercises or home treatments that I want you to use require the assistance of another person. I've also found that having the interest and caring of another individual boosts your will to keep going during struggling times in a healing cycle.

Support Groups Make a Difference

Support groups bring together people suffering from the same disease or type of trauma. Within the group, members share experiences and feelings, which may yield great mental health benefits and perhaps even boost their immune systems. Alcoholics Anonymous, for instance, began in 1935 to help people stop drinking and is one of the best-known support groups. Today there are support groups for most kinds of physical illnesses, plus a variety of mental or emotional issues—you'll find groups based on everything from cancer and heart disease to anorexia and bulimia to fibromyalgia and grief.

Support groups typically meet on a regular basis. Some are temporary, following a particular incident or trauma, while most are ongoing. Members decide to continue or stop depending on their needs. Some groups are led by mental health professionals, while others are led by lay people with experience with the particular issue.

We're almost at the end of our trail together, but it's just the beginning of your path of knowledge and treatment using Oriental Medicine. The last chapter, "And Then There Was You—Taking Charge," is perhaps the most important one in the entire book. Please take a moment to read through it. It is my wish that this book will help you find a better way to health and happiness.

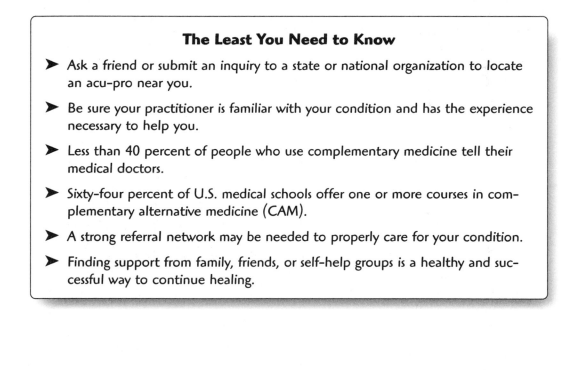

The Least You Need to Know

➤ Ask a friend or submit an inquiry to a state or national organization to locate an acu-pro near you.

➤ Be sure your practitioner is familiar with your condition and has the experience necessary to help you.

➤ Less than 40 percent of people who use complementary medicine tell their medical doctors.

➤ Sixty-four percent of U.S. medical schools offer one or more courses in complementary alternative medicine (CAM).

➤ A strong referral network may be needed to properly care for your condition.

➤ Finding support from family, friends, or self-help groups is a healthy and successful way to continue healing.

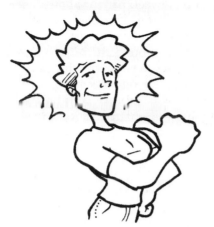

Chapter 26

And Then There Was You—Taking Charge

In This Chapter

➤ Learn to have an effective partnership in healing with your acu-pro

➤ Feel better by taking control of your lifestyle

➤ Find out the recommended ways to reduce stress

➤ Rediscover fun and laughter and the reasons why you need a daily dose of humor

➤ Enjoy the benefits of balance

Increased feelings of empowerment, self-assurance, and awareness are just a few of the benefits of a balanced healing process. I tell my patients that I believe my role in their healing is as a guide, adviser, and cheerleader, but in the end, it's *them* who make the greatest difference in their lives. I've spent a whole book filling you in on the great attributes of Oriental Medicine. However, I will remind you here that your own view of the world and the way you live life will have the greatest long-term impact on your health.

This chapter prepares you to gladly take control of your life and soar. It's been great flying with you!

Responsibility: A New Point of View

The days when you go see a medical provider to have something "done to you" are quickly vanishing. The tide has turned, and now we're all working toward creating an

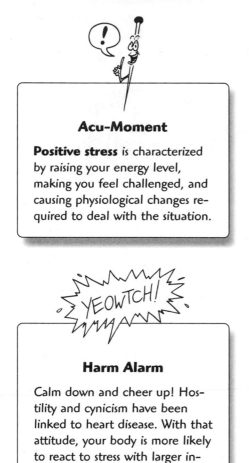

Acu-Moment

Positive stress is characterized by raising your energy level, making you feel challenged, and causing physiological changes required to deal with the situation.

Harm Alarm

Calm down and cheer up! Hostility and cynicism have been linked to heart disease. With that attitude, your body is more likely to react to stress with larger increases in heart rate, blood pressure, and stress hormones.

effective partnership between patient and provider. More patients are asking me what they can do to help themselves feel better. Chances are, since you're reading this book, you're also willing and able to take more control over your own health. Maybe you've also been taking workshops, learning how to cook differently to improve your health, and making other lifestyle changes. Put some *positive stress* to work for you by getting excited about the possibilities.

The best results in treating any condition come from a combined effort between practitioner and patient. As you've read, Oriental Medicine has taken this approach for centuries. I think it's wonderful that we're here at this time in history when it's actually become popular to take charge of your health. I can only do so much to assist you, and I need your help in order for our treatments to have lasting benefits.

Build awareness about what's going on in your life; monitor your health and reactions to certain events. As your symptoms dwindle and disappear, you will be making a transition from the healthcare that I provide to the self-care that you maintain in your life. When symptoms appear, your body is already in a little crisis. Learn how to prevent conditions from recurring, perhaps by modifying your lifestyle habits. It's your life, and I know you're up to it!

Lifestyle: It's All in Your Hands

Your acu-pro may see you for an hour or two of treatment throughout the course of your week. Do you think what you do the other 6 days and 23 hours has any impact on your condition? You bet. Working as a team, you and your acu-pro can do most anything, and modifying an out-of-balance lifestyle may be your best contribution. I advise my patients to take it slow. Getting well is not a horse race. I will go over a patient's habits to look for ways that he or she can better serve the healing process. I want to make sure that the time, energy, and money that my patients spend on healthcare are a good investment.

Healthful Lifestyle Tips

Just to get you started, here are a few of my favorite tips that I give to my stressed-out patients to aid in their healing and improve their overall health:

➤ Listen to music or read.

➤ Write down all the things that you're grateful for that day.

➤ Ask for help when you need it.

➤ Attend a play, lecture, or the symphony on a regular basis.

➤ Play sports, exercise, or stretch.

➤ Pray, meditate, and do yoga or Tai Chi.

➤ Get a hobby that fascinates you.

➤ Look at the bright side of things.

➤ Go outdoors; enjoy nature.

➤ Allow yourself to laugh or play.

➤ Get a massage.

➤ Get enough sleep.

➤ Organize your environment.

➤ Face the truth.

➤ Take a vacation or weekend getaway.

➤ Talk it over with a friend.

➤ Meet new friends who share common interests.

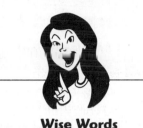

Wise Words

Laughter is good medicine. Psychoneuroimmunologists (whew, big word!) study the way our state of mind affects our health. Laughter has been found to release the same beneficial brain neurotransmitters and hormones as exercise does for the physical body. A positive outlook is good for your health!

Fun and Laughter: Remember Us?

When is the last time you had a good laugh? I mean a time when something struck you as being so funny that you lost all inhibitions, forgot totally about where you were, and let out a loud, rolling, tears-streaming, belly laugh? I bet you smile and chuckle just thinking about it. According to research at the Loma Linda University Medical School, the average adult laughs approximately 15 times per day. The average child laughs 400 times a day! As we grew up, we left a few hundred laughs a day behind us. Have we made our adult world too serious?

The same medical researchers found that laughter stimulates the immune system. Humor and exercise trigger similar physiological processes. The study group that laughed a lot, known as the laughter group, showed increased levels of good hormones, such as endorphins and neurotransmitters, and decreased levels of stress hormones, including cortisol and adrenaline. Laughter is our body's safety valve that

251

opens to counterbalance tension. Research shows that after we laugh, the elevated levels of stress hormones go back to normal, allowing our body to function smoothly and efficiently. Try it … you'll even get to keep your grin and use it again and again!

Balance and Peace of Mind

For me, it's all about freedom. I think of wellness as having the freedom to choose a life calling and a mode of self-expression that leads to passion and fulfillment. Some of the greatest joys in my life have been experienced watching patients use their new-found freedom. Imagine what you would do differently in your life if you were free of pain, your child was healthy, or you experienced peace of mind? I can tell you it's a marvel to behold patients creating a new life around their wellness, instead of building walls around a disease. Will life suddenly become easy? Well, maybe at least easier.

Your newfound balance will enable you to better handle and rebound from the challenges and growth opportunities that come along with being alive. Acu-points and Oriental Medicine are great tools to assist you in regaining your balance and peace of mind. I wish you a successful, joyful journey to wellness.

The Least You Need to Know

➤ The best results in healing come from a good partnership between patient and practitioner.

➤ Losing hostility and cynicism can be good for your heart.

➤ Build healthful habits such as exercising, listening to music, playing, and having a positive outlook.

➤ Laughter releases beneficial brain chemicals and reduces bad stress hormones.

➤ Enjoy your freedom in health to create passion and fulfillment in living.

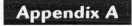

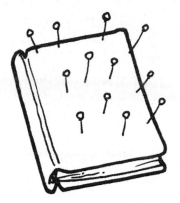

Glossary

abdominal diagnosis   Many Qi channels cross over your belly, and gentle pressure applied to specific areas will help confirm your practitioner's thoughts about your condition.

acu-points   The Chinese meaning of *acupuncture point* is the combination of the words "hole" and "position." These points serve as external doors, or openings, to the channels that access the internal muscles and organs of your body.

acupressure   The gentle but firm stimulation of acu-points by fingers, thumbs, elbows, and even feet. They are the same points along the energy channels that are used in acupuncture, but this technique forgoes the use of needles.

acupuncture   Practiced medical treatment that is over 5,000 years old. Very basically, acupuncture is the insertion of very fine needles, sometimes in conjunction with electrical stimulus, on the body's surface in order to influence physiological functioning of the body.

acupuncture needles   High-quality surgical stainless steel needles inserted into the skin that access the Qi channels in the body; these medical instruments are safe, strong, and as thin as a strand of hair.

bioelectric flow   The use of very small electrical impulses through the acupuncture needles. This method is generally used for analgesia (pain relief or prevention).

biomagnetic flow   The practice of placing biomagnets on the acu-points and measuring the microcurrents in the nerves that increase blood flow.

bronze man   An early tool used to study acupuncture points. The figure was made of bronze and had 361 holes plugged with wax to represent the location of acu-points. The man was filled with water and dressed. The student was asked to find a point and insert a needle. If the location was wrong, the needle hit metal, but if it was correct, water spurted out.

cupping   Method of stimulating acupuncture points by applying suction with a metal, wood, or glass jar, in which a partial vacuum has been created. This technique produces blood concentration at the site, and therefore stimulates it.

energy channels   A series of invisible pipes, canals, or even hallways that lead from your skin and connect to every tissue and organ inside your body.

finger measurements   Your finger's size will proportionally match your own body. To help others locate their acu-points, take into account the difference in finger width.

five-element acupuncture   Uses the five elements of wood, fire, earth, metal, and water to relate not only to symptoms but also to how your body changes according to the relationships of the elements.

healthcare   The assistance of a practitioner who uses his or her training and experience to aid you in achieving optimum physical and mental condition with the help of various tools and techniques.

herbal medicine   A complete system of diagnosis and treatment using plants, minerals, and traditionally some animals and insects to assist patients with complex medical conditions.

Japanese acupuncture   This treatment is similar to the principles of Chinese medicine, but great emphasis is placed on the abdominal exam.

medical Qi Gong   A combination of slow, easy-to-perform breathing exercises to assist a wide variety of health concerns.

moxibustion   The treatment of diseases by applying heat to acupuncture points. Acupuncture and moxibustion are considered complementary forms of treatment, and are commonly used together. Moxibustion is used for ailments such as bronchial asthma, bronchitis, certain types of paralysis, and arthritic disorders.

pulse diagnosis   In Oriental Medicine, clues to the condition of your channels that run over your body and their corresponding organs can be found by measuring your heart rate.

reflexology   Treatment method involving the stimulation of the soles of the feet and regions of the ankle joints. Many conditions of the internal organs can be treated in this manner.

self-care   Education and instruction offered by a practitioner to help you make lifestyle changes that will either speed up your healing or keep you on track.

shiatsu   A Japanese word meaning "finger pressure." This technique uses varying degrees of pressure to balance the life energy that flows through specific pathways (meridians) in the body, and relieves many chronic and acute conditions manifesting on both physical and emotional levels.

therapeutic magnets   Used in Oriental Medicine to set up specific patterns of Qi flow, capitalizing on its bioelectrical and magnetic properties. Also known as *bio-magnets*.

traditional Chinese medicine (TCM)   A medical practice that incorporates a variety of highly effective therapies into a medical system that takes each individual into account as a whole entity, rather than simply treating "diseases."

Tui-Na   Literally means "Chinese Therapeutic Massage." A physical expression of the flow of Qi energy stimulated by one person on another through various strokes applied to acu-points, channels, and muscle groups.

unit measurements   A systematic measurement of each part of the body used to locate acu-points relative to the physical proportions of the individual.

Further Reading

Classical Chinese Medicine

Unschuld, Paul. *Medicine in China: A History of Pharmaceutics*. University of California Press, 1986.

———. *Medicine in China: A History of Ideas*. University of California Press, 1988.

Veith, Ilza. *Yellow Emperor's Classic of Internal Medicine*. University of California Press, 1966.

Zhen, Li Shi, translated by Hoc Ku Huynh and Garry Seifert. *Pulse Diagnosis*. Paradigm Publications, 1985.

TCM: Traditional Chinese Medicine

Flaws, Bob. *Handbook of TCM Pediatrics*. Blue Poppy Press, 1996.

Maciocia, Giovanni. *Foundations of Chinese Medicine*. Churchill Livingstone, 1989.

———. *Practice of Chinese Medicine*. Churchill Livingstone, 1994.

———. *Tongue Diagnosis in Chinese Medicine*. Eastland Press, 1995.

Acupuncture

Bensky, Dan, and John O'Connor. *Acupuncture: A Comprehensive Text*. Eastland Press, 1981.

Birch, Stephen, and Richard Hammerschlag, Ph.D. *Acupuncture Efficacy: A Summary of Controlled Clinical Trials*. The National Academy of Acupuncture and Oriental Medicine, 1996.

Connelly, Dianne M. *Traditional Acupuncture: The Law of the Five Elements*. The Centre for Traditional Acupuncture, Inc., 1994.

Legge, David. *Close to the Bone: The Treatment of Musculoskeletal Disorder with Acupuncture and Other Traditional Chinese Medicine*. Sydney College Press, 1997.

Matsumoto, Kiiko, and Stephen Birch. *Extraordinary Vessels*. Paradigm Publications, 1986.

———. *Hara Diagnosis: Reflections on the Sea*. Paradigm Publications, 1988.

Mehta, Arun J. *Common Musculoskeletal Problems*. Hanley and Belfus, Inc., 1997.

Acupuncture: Related Titles

Chirali, Ilkay. *Cupping Therapy: Traditional Chinese Medicine*. Churchill Livingstone, 1999.

Oleson, Terrence D., Ph.D., *Auriculotherapy Manual: Chinese and Western Systems for Ear Acupuncture*. Health Care Alternatives, 1996.

Eastern Healing Arts

Flaws, Bob. *Prince Wen Hui's Cook: Chinese Dietary Therapy*. Paradigm, 1985.

Lu, Henry C. *Chinese System of Food Cures*. Sterling Publications, 1986.

Eastern Energetic Arts

Yang, Jwing Ming. *Eight Simple Qigong Exercises*. YMAA Publications, 1997.

———. *Qigong for Arthritis*. YMAA Publications, 1997.

———. *Essence of Shaolin White Crane*. YMAA Publications, 1996.

———. *Root of Chinese QiGong*. YMAA Publications, 1997.

Bioelectric and Magnet Therapy

Becker, R.O., and Gary Selden. *Body Electric*. William Morrow & Co., 1987.

Traditional Eastern Manual Therapies

Mazunaga, Shizuto. *Zen Shiatsu*. Japan Publications, 1977.

Mochizuki, James. *Anma, Art of Japanese Massage*. Kotobuki Publications, 1999.

Sun, Chengnan. *Chinese Bodywork: Complete Manual of Therapeutic Massage*. Pacific View Press, 1993.

Innovative Bodywork Therapies

Calais-Germain, Blandine. *Anatomy of Movement Exercises*. Eastland Press, 1996.

————. *Anatomy of Movement*. Eastland Press, 1993.

Western Herbal Medicine

Ody, Penelope. *Complete Medicinal Herbal*. Dorling Kindersley, 1993.

Nutrition, Naturopathy, Natural Medicine

Balch, James, and Phyllis Balch. *Prescription for Nutritional Healing*. Avery Pub Group, 1996.

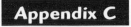

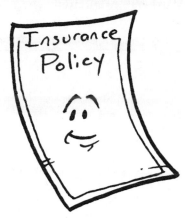

Insurance Coverage

I am always asked if insurance companies cover acupuncture. As you can see from the following chart, we've got a ways to go. In many states, we have no mandatory insurance coverage for acupuncture. Parity means that if insurance carriers pay for another health professional to perform acupuncture therapy, then they must pay the acupuncturist who is also qualified to deliver this therapy.

State	Mandated Third-Party Reimbursement	Mandated Workers' Compensation Reimbursement	Mandated Professional Liability Insurance
Alaska	No	No	No disclosure required
Arizona	No	No	No
Arkansas	No	No	No
California	Parity	Yes	No
Colorado	No	No	Yes
Connecticut	No	No	No
D.C.	No	No	No
Florida	Parity	No	Yes
Hawaii	No	No	No
Illinois	No	No	No
Iowa	No	No	No
Louisiana	N/A	N/A	N/A
Maine	Parity	No	No
Maryland	No	No	No

State	Mandated Third-Party Reimbursement	Mandated Workers' Compensation Reimbursement	Mandated Professional Liability Insurance
Massachusetts	No	No	No
Minnesota	No	No	No
Missouri	No	No	No
Montana	Yes	Yes	No
Nevada	Yes	Yes	No
New Hampshire	No	No	No
New Jersey	No	No	No
New Mexico	No	No	No
New York	No	No	No
N. Carolina	No	No	No
Oregon	Parity	Yes	Yes
Pennsylvania	No	No	No
Rhode Island	No	No	No
S. Carolina	No	No	No
Texas	No	No	No
Utah	No	No	No
Vermont	No	No	No
Virginia	No	No	No
Washington	Yes	No	No
West Virginia	Yes	Yes	No
Wisconsin	No	No	No

Footnote: Used with permission of Acupuncture and Oriental Medicine Laws, *by Barbara B. Mitchell, L.Ac. (National Acupuncture Foundation, 1999)*

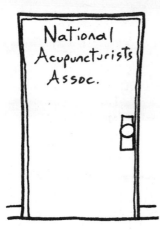

State and National Organizations

For more information about acupuncture and acupressure, including help finding the best Oriental Medical health team in your area, contact the following organizations:

Accreditation Commission for Acupuncture and Oriental Medicine (ACAOM)
1010 Wayne Ave., Suite 1270
Silver Spring, MD 20910
301-608-9680; fax 301-608-9576

Acupressure Institute
1533 Shattuck Ave.
Berkeley, CA 94709
415-845-1059

AIDS and Chinese Medicine Institute
455 Arkansas St.
San Francisco, CA 94107
415-282-4028; fax 415-282-2935

American Academy of Medical Acupuncture (AAMA) and Medical Acupuncture Research Foundation (MARF)
5820 Wilshire Blvd., Suite 500
Los Angeles, CA 90036
213-937-5514; fax 213-937-0059

American Association of Oriental Medicine (AAOM)
433 Front St.
Catasauqua, PA 18032
610-266-1433; fax 610-264-2768

American Association for Teachers in Oriental Medicine
P.O. Box 9563
Austin, TX 78766-9563
512-451-2866
acuaoma@aol.com

American Oriental Bodywork Therapy Association (AOBTA)
Glenndale Executive Campus, Suite 510
1000 White Horse Rd.
Voorhees, NJ 08043
609-782-1616; fax 609-782-1653

Council of Colleges of Acupuncture and Oriental Medicine (CCAOM)
1010 Wayne Ave., Suite 1270
Silver Spring, MD 20910
301-608-9175; fax 301-608-9576
www.ccaom.org

International Veterinary Acupuncture Society
268 West Third St., #4
P.O. Box 2074
303-258-3767

NAFTA Acupuncture and Oriental Medicine Commission
14637 Starr Rd. SE
Olalla, WA 98359
253-851-6896; fax 253-851-6883

National Academy of Acupuncture and Oriental Medicine
P.O. Box 62
Tarrytown, NY 10591
914-631-2369

**National Acupuncture and Oriental Medicine Alliance
(Acupuncture Alliance)**
14637 Starr Rd. SE
Olalla, WA 98359
253-851-6896; fax 253-851-6883
www.acuall.org

National Acupuncture Detoxification Association (NADA)
c/o NADA Literature Clearinghouse
P.O. Box 1927
Vancouver, WA 98668-1927
360-260-8620 (fax or phone)

National Acupuncture Foundation (NAF)
P.O. Box 2271
Gig Harbor, WA 98335-4271
253-851-6538; fax 253-851-6883

National Certification Commission for Acupuncture and Oriental Medicine (NCCAOM)
11 Canal Center Plaza, Suite 300
Alexandria, VA 22314
703-548-9004; fax 703-548-9079

National Sports Acupuncture Association
1237 Siskiyou, #130
Ashland, OR 97520
415-704-3123

Society for Acupuncture Research (SAR)
4733 Bethesda Ave., Suite 804
Bethesda, MD 20814
fax 202-363-3859

International Academy of Advanced Reflexology and Advanced Reflexology Complementary Health Center
704 Decatur St.
Bethlehem, PA 18017-4808
1-800-221-7963; local 610-882-1112; fax 610-866-1333

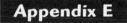

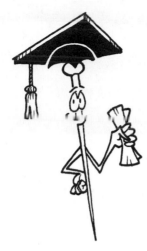

Acupuncture Schools

The following is a listing of the accredited programs in this country where you could either go to school if so inspired, take a class, or find a qualified practitioner.

Accreditation Commission for Acupuncture and Oriental Medicine (ACAOM)

1010 Wayne Ave., Suite 1270
Silver Spring, MD 20910
301-608-9680; fax 301-608-9576

The Accreditation Commission for Acupuncture and Oriental Medicine (ACAOM), formerly the National Accreditation Commission for Schools and Colleges of Acupuncture and Oriental Medicine (NACSCAOM), was established in June 1982 by the Council of Colleges of Acupuncture and Oriental Medicine (CCAOM). Its mission is to foster excellence in acupuncture and Oriental Medicine education. The commission acts as an independent body to evaluate first-professional Master's degree and professional Master's level certificate and diploma programs in acupuncture, and first-professional Master's degree and professional Master's level certificate and diploma programs in Oriental Medicine with a concentration in both acupuncture and herbal therapies for a level of performance, integrity, and quality that entitles the practitioners to the confidence of the educational community and the public they serve. The commission is the sole accrediting agency recognized by the U.S. Department of Education and the Council on Higher Education Accreditation to accredit professional programs in the field. ACAOM is also a charter member of the Association of Specialized and Profes-sional Accreditors.

Accredited Programs

** Academy for Five Element Acupuncture

"Licentiate of Acupuncture" program

> 1170-A E. Hallandale Beach Blvd.
> Hallandale, FL 33009
> 954-456-6336; fax 954-456-3944
> E-mail: AFEA@compuserve.com
> Web site: www.acupuncturist.com
> Accredited: 5/98; next review: Spring 2001

* Academy of Chinese Culture and Health Sciences

"Master of Science in Traditional Chinese Medicine" program

> 1601 Clay St.
> Oakland, CA 94612
> 510-763-7787; fax 510-834-8646
> E-mail: acchs@best.com
> Web site: www.acchs.edu
> Accredited: 11/92; reaccredited: 11/97; next review: Fall 2001

** Academy of Chinese Healing Arts

"Diploma in Oriental Medicine" program

> 505 South Orange Ave.
> Sarasota, FL 34236
> 941-955-4456; fax 941-365-6758
> E-mail: acha@gte.net
> Web site: www.acha.net
> Accredited: 11/99; next review: Fall 2003

* Academy of Oriental Medicine at Austin

"Master of Science in Oriental Medicine" program

> 2700 West Anderson Lane, Suite 117
> Austin, TX 78757
> 512-454-1188; fax 512-454-7001
> E-mail: acuaoma@aol.com
> Web site: www.aoma.edu
> Accredited: 11/96; next review: Fall 2000

* American College of Acupuncture and Oriental Medicine

"Master of Science in Oriental Medicine" program

> 9100 Park West Dr.
> Houston, TX 77063
> 713-780-9777; fax 713-781-5781
> E-mail: 102657.1730@compuserve.com
> Web site: www.acaom.edu
> Accredited: 5/96; reaccredited: 5/99; next review: Spring 2003

* American College of Traditional Chinese Medicine

"Master of Science in Traditional Chinese Medicine" program

> 455 Arkansas St.
> San Francisco, CA 94107
> 415-282-7600; fax 415-282-0856
> E-mail: lhuang@actcm.org
> Web site: www.actcm.org
> Accredited: 11/91; reaccredited: 11/96; next review: Fall 2001

** Atlantic Institute of Oriental Medicine

"Diploma in Traditional Chinese Medicine" program

> 1057 SE 17th St.
> Fort Lauderdale, FL 33316-2116
> 954-463-3888; fax 954-463-3878
> E-mail: atom3@ix.netcom.com
> Web site: www.khuang.com/atom
> Accredited: 5/99; next review: Spring 2002

* Bastyr University

"Master of Science in Acupuncture" program
"Master of Science in Acupuncture and Oriental Medicine" program

> 14500 Juanita Dr., NE
> Kenmore, WA 98028
> 425-823-1300; fax 425-823-6222
> E-mail: admiss@bastyr.edu
> Web site: www.bastyr.edu
> Accredited: 11/94; reaccredited: 11/99; next review: Fall 2004

* Dongguk Royal University

"Master of Science in Oriental Medicine" program

> 440 South Shatto Pl.
> Los Angeles, CA 90020
> 213-487-0110; fax 213-487-0527
> E-mail: dru@pdc.net
> Web site: www.dru.edu
> Accredited: 5/94; reaccredited: 5/99; next review: Spring 2002

* Emperor's College of Traditional Oriental Medicine

"Master of Traditional Oriental Medicine" program

> 1807 B. Wilshire Blvd.
> Santa Monica, CA 90403
> 310-453-8300; fax 310-829-3838
> E-mail: dsl@emperors.edu
> Web site: www.emperors.edu
> Accredited: 5/89; reaccredited: 11/94, 5/98; next review: Spring 2001

* Five Branches Institute: College of Traditional Chinese Medicine

"Master of Traditional Chinese Medicine" program

> 200 7th Ave.
> Santa Cruz, CA 95062
> 831-476-9424; fax 831-476-8928
> E-mail: tcm@fivebranches.edu
> Web site: www.fivebranches.edu
> Accredited: 5/96; reaccredited: 5/99; next review: Spring 2003

** Florida Institute of Traditional Chinese Medicine

"Diploma in Traditional Chinese Medicine" program

> 5335 66th St. N.
> St. Petersburg, FL 33709
> 727-546-6565; fax 727-547-0703
> E-mail: fitcm@gte.net
> Web site: www.fitcm.com
> Accredited: 11/99; next review: Fall 2002

* International Institute of Chinese Medicine

"Master of Oriental Medicine" program

> P.O. Box 4991
> Santa Fe, NM 87502
> 505-473-5233, 1-800-377-4561; fax 505-473-9279
> E-mail: 102152.3463@compuserve.com
> Web site: www.thuntek.net/iicm
> ** Branch:*
> 4600 Montgomery, NE, Bldg. 1, Ste.1
> Albuquerque, NM 87109
> 505-883-5569; fax 505-883-5569
> E-mail: panda@thuntek.net
> Accredited: 11/90; reaccredited: 11/95; next review: Fall 2000

** Maryland Institute of Traditional Chinese Medicine

"Diploma in Acupuncture" program

> 4641 Montgomery Ave., Suite 415
> Bethesda, MD 20814
> 301-718-7373; fax 301-718-0735
> E-mail: martindell@aol.com
> Web site: www.mitcm.org
> Accredited: 5/98; next review: Spring 2001

* Meiji College of Oriental Medicine

"Master of Science in Oriental Medicine" program

> 2550 Shattuck Ave.
> Berkeley, CA 94704
> 510-666-8248; fax 510-666-0111
> E-mail: meiji@pacbell.net
> Accredited: 5/98; next review: Spring 2002

* Midwest College of Oriental Medicine

"Certificate of Completion in Acupuncture" program
"Master of Science in Oriental Medicine" program

> 6226 Bankers Rd., Suites 5 & 6
> Racine, WI 53403
> 414-554-2010; fax 414-554-7475
> E-mail: info@acupuncture.edu
> Web site: www.acupuncture.edu
> Accredited: 11/93; reaccredited: 11/98; next review: Fall 2001

** Minnesota Institute of Acupuncture and Herbal Studies

"Diploma in Acupuncture" program
"Diploma in Oriental Medicine" program

> Northwestern Health Sciences University
> West 84th Street
> Bloomington, MN 55431
> 612-888-4777; fax 612-887-1398
> E-mail: miahs@nwhealth.edu
> Web site: www.nwhealth.edu
> Accredited: 5/99; next review: Spring 2002

* National College of Oriental Medicine

"Master of Oriental Medicine" program

> 7100 Lake Ellenor Dr.
> Orlando, FL 32809
> 407-888-8689; fax 407-888-8211
> E-mail: info@acupunctureschool.com
> Web site: www.acupunctureschool.com
> Accredited: 11/97; next review: Fall 2000

* New England School of Acupuncture

"Master of Acupuncture" program

> 40 Belmont St.
> Watertown, MA 02472
> 617-926-1788; fax 617-924-4167
> Web site: www.nesa.edu
> Accredited: 2/88; reaccredited: 11/93, 11/98; next review: Fall 2003

* New York College for Holistic Health Education and Research

"Master of Science in Acupuncture" program
"Master of Science in Oriental Medicine" program

> 6801 Jericho Turnpike
> Syosset, NY 11791-4465
> 516-364-0808; fax 516-364-0989
> E-mail: nycinfo@nycollege.edu
> Web site: www.nycollege.edu
> Accredited: 11/96; next review: Fall 2000

* Northwest Institute of Acupuncture and Oriental Medicine

"Master of Acupuncture" program
"Master of Traditional Chinese Medicine" program

> 701 N. 34th St., Suite 300
> Seattle, WA 98103
> 206-633-2419; fax 206-633-5578
> E-mail: folks@niaom.edu
> Web site: www.niaom.cdu
> Accredited: 4/90; reaccredited: 5/95; next review: Spring 2000

* Oregon College of Oriental Medicine

"Master of Acupuncture and Oriental Medicine" program

> 10525 SE Cherry Blossom Dr.
> Portland, OR 97216
> 503-253-3443; fax 503-253-2701
> E-mail: 103226.164@compuserve.com
> Web site: www.infinite.org/oregon.acupuncture
> Accredited: 5/89; reaccredited: 5/94, 5/99; next review: Spring 2004

* Pacific College of Oriental Medicine

"Master of Science in Traditional Oriental Medicine" program

> 7445 Mission Valley Rd., Suites 103–106
> San Diego, CA 92108
> 619-574-6909; fax 619-574-6641
> E-mail: jmiller@ormed.edu
> Web site: www.ormed.edu
> * Branch:
> *"Master of Science in Acupuncture" program*
> *"Master of Science in Oriental Medicine" program*
> 915 Broadway, 3rd Floor
> New York, NY 10010
> 212-982-3456; fax 212-982-6514
> Accredited: 11/90; reaccredited: 11/95; next review: Fall 2000

* Samra University of Oriental Medicine

"Master of Science in Oriental Medicine" program

> 3000 South Robertson Blvd., 4th Floor
> Los Angeles, CA 90034
> 310-202-6444; fax 310-202-6007
> E-mail: admissions@samra.edu
> Web site: www.samra.edu
> Accredited: 10/89; reaccredited: 11/94, 11/99; next review: Fall 2003

* Santa Barbara College of Oriental Medicine

"Master of Acupuncture and Oriental Medicine" program

> 1919 State St., Suite 204
> Santa Barbara, CA 93101
> 805-898-1180; fax 805-682-1864
> E-mail: admissions@SBCOM.edu
> Web site: www.SBCOM.edu
> Accredited: 5/95; reaccredited 5/98; next review: Spring 2002

* Seattle Institute of Oriental Medicine

"Master of Acupuncture and Oriental Medicine" program

> 916 NE 65th St., Suite B
> Seattle, WA 98115
> 206-517-4541; fax 206-526-1932
> E-mail: info@siom.com
> Web site: www.siom.com
> Accredited: 5/98; next review: Spring 2001

* South Baylo University

"Master of Science in Acupuncture and Oriental Medicine" program

> 1126 N. Brookhurst St.
> Anaheim, CA 92801
> 714-533-1495; fax 714-533-6040
> E-mail: ron@southbaylo.edu
> Web site: www.southbaylo.edu
> ** Branch:*
> 2727 W. 6th St.
> Los Angeles, CA 90015
> 213-738-0712; fax 213-480-1332
> Accredited: 6/93; reaccredited: 11/96; next review: Spring 2000

* Southwest Acupuncture College
"Master of Science in Oriental Medicine" program

> 2960 Rodeo Park Dr. West
> Santa Fe, NM 87505
> 505-438-8884; fax 505-438-8883
> E-mail: 105315.3010@compuserve.com
> Web site: www.swacupuncture.com
> * *Branch:*
> 4308 Carlisle NE, Suite 205
> Albuquerque, NM 87107
> 505-888-8898; fax 505-888-1380
> * *Branch:*
> 6658 Gunpark Dr.
> Boulder, CO 80301
> 303-581-9955; fax 303-581-9944
> Accredited: 10/89; reaccredited: 5/95; next review: Spring 2000

** Swedish Institute: School of Acupuncture and Oriental Studies
"Diploma in Acupuncture" program

> 226 West 26th St.
> New York, NY 10001
> 212-924-5900; fax 212-924-7600
> Web site: www.swedish-institute.com
> Accredited: 5/99; next review: Spring 2002

* Tai Hsuan Foundation: College of Acupuncture and Herbal Medicine
"Master of Acupuncture and Oriental Medicine" program

> 2600 S. King St., #206
> Honolulu, HI 96826
> 1-800-942-4788; fax 808-947-1152
> E-mail: taihsuancollege@cs.com
> Web site: acupuncture-hi.com
> Accredited: 4/91; reaccredited: 5/96; next review: Spring 2000

* Texas College of Traditional Chinese Medicine

"Master of Science in Oriental Medicine" program

> 4005 Manchaca Rd., Suite 200
> Austin, TX 78704
> 512-444-8082; fax 512-444-6345
> E-mail: texastcm@texastcm.edu
> Web site: www.texastcm.edu
> Accredited: 11/96; next review: Fall 2000

* Traditional Acupuncture Institute

"Master of Acupuncture" program

> 10227 Wincopin Circle, Suite 100
> Columbia, MD 21044-3422
> 301-596-6006; fax 410-964-3544
> E-mail: admissions@tai.edu
> Web site: www.tai.edu
> Accredited: 5/85; reaccredited: 11/90, 11/95; next review: Fall 2000

* Tri-State College of Acupuncture

"Master of Science in Acupuncture" program

> 80 8th Ave., 4th Floor
> New York, NY 10011
> 212-242-2255; fax 212-242-2920
> E-mail: TSITCA@aol.com
> Accredited: 11/93; reaccredited: 11/98; next review: Fall 2003

* Yo San University of Traditional Chinese Medicine

"Master of Acupuncture and Traditional Chinese Medicine" program

> 1314 Second St., Suite 200
> Santa Monica, CA 90401
> 310-917-2202; fax 310-917-2203
> E-mail: info@yosan.edu
> Web site: www.Yosan.edu
> Accredited: 5/93; reaccredited 5/98; next review: Spring 2003

Candidate Programs

** Acupressure-Acupuncture Institute

"Diploma in Oriental Medicine" program

> 10506 North Kendall Dr.
> Miami, FL 33176
> 305-595-9500; fax 305-595-2622
> E-mail: aai@acupuncture.pair.com
> Web site: www.acupuncture.pair.com
> Candidacy granted: 5/98

*China International Medical University

"Master of Science in Traditional Chinese Medicine" program

> 822 South Robertson Blvd., Suite 300
> Los Angeles, CA 90035
> 310-289-8394, fax 310-289-0306
> E-mail: cimu@worldnet.att.net
> Web site: home.att.net/~cimu/
> Candidacy granted: 11/99

** Dallas Institute of Acupuncture and Oriental Medicine

"Diploma in Oriental Medicine" program

> 2947 Walnut Hill Lane, Suite 101
> Dallas, TX 75229
> 214-350-4282; fax 214-350-9056
> E-mail: diaom@flash.net
> Candidacy granted: 5/99

* Mercy College: Program in Acupuncture and Oriental Medicine

"Master of Professional Studies in Acupuncture and Oriental Medicine" program

> 555 Broadway
> Dobbs Ferry, NY 10522
> 914-674-7401; fax 914-674-7374
> E-mail: acu@mercynet.edu
> Web site: www.mercynet.edu/programs/graduate/acupuncture
> Candidacy granted: 11/97

* National College of Naturopathic Medicine

"Master of Science in Oriental Medicine" program

> 1049 S.W. Porter
> Portland, OR 97201
> 503-499-4343; fax 503-499-0022
> E-mail: admissions@ncnm.edu
> Web site: www.ncnm.edu
> Candidacy granted: 11/97

** New York Institute of Chinese Medicine

"Diploma in Acupuncture" program

> 155 First St.
> Mineola, NY 11501
> 516-739-2798; fax 516-739-2798
> Candidacy granted: 11/99

** Traditional Chinese Medical College of Hawaii

"Diploma in Oriental Medicine" program

> P.O. Box 2288
> Kamuela, HI 96743
> 808-885-9226 (fax also)
> E-mail: chinese@ilhawaii.com
> Web site: www.ilhawaii.net/~chinese
> Candidacy granted: 5/96

* *A first-professional master's degree program.*

** *A first-professional master's level certificate or diploma program.*

Index

C

U–V

W–X

Y–Z

Check Out These
Best-Selling
COMPLETE IDIOT'S GUIDES®

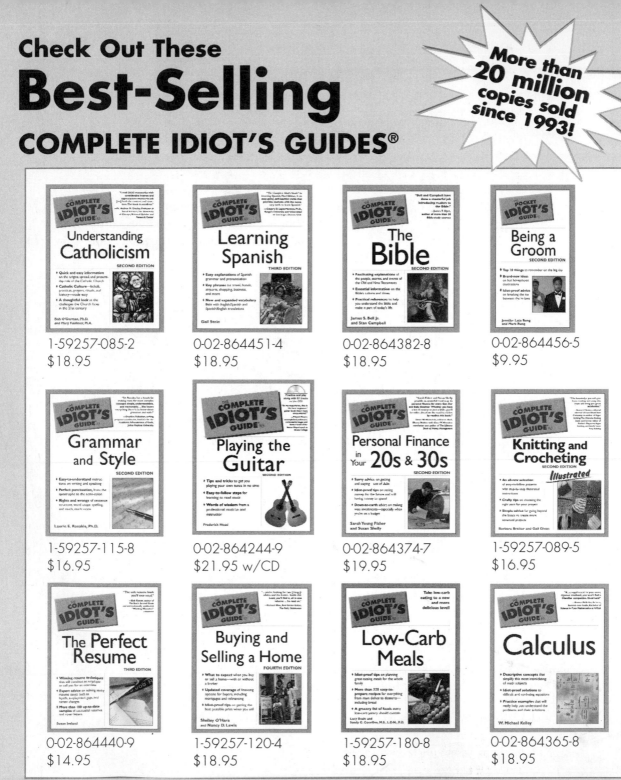

Understanding **Catholicism**
SECOND EDITION

1-59257-085-2
$18.95

Learning **Spanish**
THIRD EDITION

0-02-864451-4
$18.95

The **Bible**
SECOND EDITION

0-02-864382-8
$18.95

Being a **Groom**
SECOND EDITION

0-02-864456-5
$9.95

Grammar and **Style**
SECOND EDITION

1-59257-115-8
$16.95

Playing the **Guitar**
SECOND EDITION

0-02-864244-9
$21.95 w/CD

Personal Finance in Your **20s & 30s**
SECOND EDITION

0-02-864374-7
$19.95

Knitting and Crocheting
SECOND EDITION
Illustrated

1-59257-089-5
$16.95

The **Perfect Resume**
THIRD EDITION

0-02-864440-9
$14.95

Buying and Selling a Home
FOURTH EDITION

1-59257-120-4
$18.95

Low-Carb Meals

1-59257-180-8
$18.95

Calculus

0-02-864365-8
$18.95

More than *450 titles* in *30 different categories*
Available at booksellers everywhere

ALPHA